INTRODUCTION

Osteoporosis, a familiar yet often overlooked condition, stands as a significant public health concern worldwide. This skeletal disorder is characterized by a bone mass and density deterioration, resulting in increased fragility and susceptibility to fractures. As bones become porous and brittle, the risk of fractures, particularly in the spine, hip, and wrist, escalates. Osteoporosis predominantly affects older adults, particularly postmenopausal women, but it can also impact men and individuals of all ages. Recognizing the multifaceted nature of this condition, where genetic, hormonal, and lifestyle factors intersect, offers a crucial foundation for developing effective preventive strategies.

One pivotal aspect in managing and preventing osteoporosis is the role of diet. Nutrition plays a central role in bone health, influencing the attainment and maintenance of optimal bone density throughout one's life. A diet rich in specific nutrients and prudent lifestyle choices can contribute significantly to the fortification of bones and the reduction of fracture risk. In this exploration, we delve into the intricate relationship between osteoporosis and dietary practices, examining the essential nutrients that support bone health and unveiling nutritional guidelines that may mitigate the impact of this skeletal disorder.

Understanding the underlying mechanisms of osteoporosis and the influence of diet on bone metabolism is crucial for individuals seeking to manage their bone health proactively and for healthcare professionals aiming to formulate personalized dietary recommendations. This comprehensive exploration seeks to shed light on the interconnectedness of osteoporosis and diet, providing insights into the nutritional strategies that may serve as powerful tools in preventing and managing this prevalent skeletal condition.

CHAPTER ONE

Definition Of Osteoporosis

Osteoporosis is a systemic skeletal disorder characterized by compromised bone density and microarchitecture, leading to increased bone fragility and a heightened risk of fractures. This condition arises when there is an imbalance in the dynamic process of bone remodelling, with bone resorption outpacing bone formation. Essentially, it results in a reduction of bone mass and a deterioration of bone quality, rendering the skeletal structure more susceptible to fractures, especially in areas such as the spine, hip, and wrist.

Explanation of the Condition:

Osteoporosis is often asymptomatic in its early stages, earning it the moniker of the "silent disease." The gradual loss of bone density occurs without apparent signs until a fracture occurs, often triggered by minor stresses or falls that would not typically cause harm in individuals with healthy bones. The primary underlying factors contributing to osteoporosis include hormonal changes, particularly in postmenopausal women who experience a decline in estrogen levels and age-related reductions in bone formation and calcium absorption. Other contributors include genetics, nutritional deficiencies, a sedentary lifestyle, and certain medical conditions or medications that can adversely affect bone health.

Impact on Bone Density and Strength:

Osteoporosis fundamentally alters the composition of bones, leading to a decrease in both bone mineral density (BMD) and the trabecular and cortical microarchitecture. Bone mineral density reflects the amount of mineral (mainly calcium and phosphorus) in bone tissue and is a crucial indicator of bone strength. In osteoporosis, the bones become porous and brittle due to a decline in mineral content, making them more prone to fractures. This compromised structural integrity results from an imbalance in the bone remodelling process, with increased bone resorption by osteoclasts (cells that break down bone) surpassing bone formation by osteoblasts (cells responsible for building new bone).

The impact of osteoporosis on bone density and strength is profound. Standard bone architecture, characterized by a delicate balance between resorption and formation, becomes disrupted. The trabecular bone, the spongy tissue at the core of bones, and the cortical bone, the dense outer layer, both undergo detrimental changes. As a consequence, bones lose their ability to withstand mechanical stress, and even minor incidents can lead to fractures. Spinal compression fractures, hip fractures, and wrist fractures are common manifestations of osteoporosis, each posing significant health risks and impairing the overall quality of life.

CAUSES AND RISK FACTORS OF OSTEOPOROSIS

Osteoporosis is a multifaceted condition influenced by a range of causes and risk factors. Understanding these factors is crucial for both prevention and effective management. Here, we explore the diverse elements contributing to osteoporosis, including ageing, gender, genetics, and lifestyle factors.

A. Aging:

1. Discussion of Age-Related Bone Loss: Age is a prominent risk factor for osteoporosis, and bone loss is a natural part of ageing. As individuals age, the balance between bone formation and resorption becomes disrupted. Osteoblasts (bone-forming cells) become less efficient, leading to a gradual reduction in bone mass. This age-related bone loss is more pronounced in women, especially after menopause, when estrogen levels decline significantly.

2. Impact on Bone Density Over Time: The cumulative effect of age-related bone loss is a decline in bone density over time. This bone mass reduction compromises bones' structural integrity, making them more susceptible to

fractures. The spine, hips, and wrists are particularly vulnerable, and fractures in these areas can have severe consequences for individuals affected by osteoporosis.

B. Gender:

1. Explanation of Higher Prevalence in Women: Osteoporosis is more prevalent in women, and this gender disparity is primarily attributed to the hormonal changes associated with menopause. Estrogen, a crucial hormone in maintaining bone density, declines significantly during menopause, leading to accelerated bone loss. Women generally reach lower peak bone mass than men, and the hormonal changes postmenopause exacerbate the risk of osteoporosis.

2. Hormonal Factors Contributing to Bone Health: Hormonal factors, particularly sex hormones like estrogen and testosterone, play a pivotal role in bone health. Estrogen, in particular, has a protective effect on bone density by inhibiting bone resorption. Reduced estrogen levels in postmenopausal women contribute significantly to the development of osteoporosis. In men, lower testosterone levels associated with ageing can also contribute to bone loss, albeit typically at a slower rate compared to women.

C. Genetics:

1. Overview of Genetic Factors Influencing Susceptibility: Genetic factors contribute substantially to an individual's susceptibility to osteoporosis. Specific genetic variations can influence bone density, bone turnover, and the overall structure of bones. Variations in genes related to collagen formation, vitamin D metabolism, and bone mineralization can impact bone

health.

2. Family History and its Role in Osteoporosis Risk: A family history of osteoporosis is a significant risk factor. If parents or siblings have a history of fractures or osteoporosis, there is an increased likelihood of a genetic predisposition. However, while genetics play a role, environmental factors and lifestyle choices also contribute to overall bone health.

D. Lifestyle Factors:

1. Importance of Physical Activity: Physical activity is crucial for maintaining bone health. Weight-bearing exercises, resistance training, and activities that stimulate bone formation help to preserve bone density. Sedentary lifestyles contribute to accelerated bone loss, emphasizing the importance of regular and varied physical activity.

2. Role of Diet in Bone Health: Adequate nutrition, especially calcium and vitamin D intake, is essential for optimal bone health. A diet rich in these nutrients supports bone formation and mineralization. Conversely, deficiencies can contribute to bone loss. Additionally, excessive intake of sodium, caffeine, and phosphoric acid (found in some sodas) may adversely affect calcium balance and bone density.

3. Connection Between Smoking and Alcohol Consumption: Smoking and excessive alcohol consumption are detrimental to bone health. Smoking interferes with the absorption of calcium, while heavy alcohol consumption can disrupt bone formation and increase the risk of fractures. Both habits contribute to accelerated bone loss, emphasizing the need for lifestyle

VICTORIA EASTERBY

modifications for the prevention of osteoporosis.

SYMPTOMS OF OSTEOPOROSIS

Osteoporosis is often referred to as the "silent disease" because it typically progresses without noticeable symptoms until a fracture occurs. The absence of early warning signs underscores the importance of proactive measures in identifying and managing this skeletal condition. Here, we explore the symptoms associated with osteoporosis and highlight the significance of early detection.

1. Fractures: The most overt symptom of osteoporosis is often the occurrence of fractures. Individuals with osteoporosis are at an increased risk of fractures, especially in weight-bearing bones such as the spine, hips, and wrists. Fractures can result from minimal trauma, and in some cases, they may occur spontaneously. Spinal compression fractures can lead to a stooped posture (kyphosis), loss of height, and chronic back pain.

2. Back Pain: Chronic back pain, particularly in the lower back, is a common symptom of osteoporosis. This pain can be attributed to vertebral fractures or collapsed vertebrae, which can occur without a specific injury or trauma. The compression of spinal nerves due to fractures may also contribute to pain and discomfort.

3. Loss of Height: Osteoporosis can lead to a gradual loss of height over time. Vertebral fractures, which often go unnoticed, may reduce overall height as the spine becomes compressed. This loss of height is more prominent in the later stages of osteoporosis and can contribute to a stooped or hunched posture.

4. Changes in Posture: Kyphosis, an exaggerated curvature of the upper back, is a characteristic change in posture associated with osteoporosis. As vertebral fractures occur, the spine may curve forward, leading to a noticeable upper back rounding. A reduction in mobility often accompanies this change in posture.

5. Decreased Grip Strength and Muscular Weakness: Osteoporosis can affect bone density and muscle strength. Individuals with osteoporosis may experience decreased grip strength and overall muscular weakness. This can contribute to an increased risk of falls and fractures.

6. Tooth Loss: In some cases, osteoporosis may affect the jawbone, leading to tooth loss. The jawbone, like other bones in the body, can experience a decrease in density, potentially compromising the stability of teeth.

DIAGNOSIS OF OSTEOPOROSIS

Diagnosing osteoporosis involves a multifaceted approach, integrating clinical assessments, imaging techniques, and bone density measurements to evaluate bone health and fracture risk. Early detection is paramount for effective management and intervention. Here, we delve into the various components of the diagnostic process for osteoporosis.

1. Clinical Assessment: Clinical evaluations are crucial in identifying individuals at risk of osteoporosis. Healthcare professionals consider factors such as age, gender, family history, medical history, and lifestyle habits. A comprehensive review of medications, particularly those that may impact bone health, is also part of the clinical assessment. Individuals reporting symptoms such as back pain, height loss, or a history of fractures may prompt further investigation.

2. Bone Mineral Density (BMD) Testing: BMD testing is a cornerstone of osteoporosis diagnosis. Dual-energy X-ray absorptiometry (DXA) is the most widely used technique for measuring bone density. DXA scans assess BMD at specific sites, typically the spine, hip, or forearm. The results are expressed as a T-score, which compares an individual's bone density to that of a healthy young adult.

A T-score of -2.5 or lower indicates osteoporosis, while a T-score between -1 and -2.5 signifies osteopenia, a condition of low bone density that precedes osteoporosis.

3. Fracture Risk Assessment: Tools like FRAX (Fracture Risk Assessment Tool) are used to estimate an individual's 10-year probability of a major osteoporotic fracture. This tool incorporates clinical risk factors, such as age, gender, previous fractures, and secondary causes of bone loss, to provide a comprehensive assessment of fracture risk. Healthcare providers use FRAX results, in conjunction with BMD measurements, to guide treatment decisions.

4. Laboratory Tests: Blood tests may be conducted to assess specific markers related to bone turnover and metabolism. Levels of markers like serum calcium, phosphorus, alkaline phosphatase, and vitamin D can provide insights into bone health. Additionally, testing for specific genetic factors related to bone metabolism may be considered in some cases.

5. Imaging Studies: While DXA remains the gold standard for bone density assessment, other imaging studies may be employed for specific situations. Quantitative computed tomography (QCT) and peripheral DXA are alternative techniques that provide additional information about bone density in particular regions.

6. Vertebral Fracture Assessment (VFA): VFA is a specialized X-ray imaging technique used to detect vertebral fractures. This assessment can be performed simultaneously with a DXA scan, offering valuable insights into the presence of fractures that might not be clinically apparent.

7. Clinical Guidelines and Recommendations: Established clinical guidelines guide the diagnosis and management of osteoporosis. These guidelines, often set forth by organizations such as the National Osteoporosis Foundation (NOF) or the World Health Organization (WHO), provide evidence-based recommendations for screening, diagnosis, and treatment based on individual risk factors and bone health assessments.

TREATMENT APPROACHES FOR OSTEOPOROSIS

Effectively managing osteoporosis involves a multifaceted approach that integrates medications, lifestyle modifications, and nutritional interventions. Tailoring treatment strategies to individual needs is crucial for optimizing outcomes and minimizing the risk of fractures. Here, we explore the critical components of treatment for osteoporosis.

A. Medications:

1. Overview of Medications for Osteoporosis: Medications play a pivotal role in the treatment of osteoporosis, aiming to enhance bone density, reduce fracture risk, and maintain skeletal integrity. Various classes of medications are available, each targeting specific aspects of bone metabolism. Commonly prescribed medications include bisphosphonates, selective estrogen receptor modulators (SERMs), hormone therapy (especially for postmenopausal women), denosumab, and anabolic agents such as teriparatide.

2. Bisphosphonates, Hormone Therapy, and Other Options:

• Bisphosphonates: These drugs, including alendronate, risedronate, and zoledronic acid, inhibit bone resorption and promote bone density. They are often prescribed for postmenopausal women and men with osteoporosis.

• Hormone Therapy: Estrogen and hormone replacement therapy may be considered for postmenopausal women to mitigate the impact of estrogen decline on bone density.

• Denosumab: This biologic agent inhibits bone resorption and is administered as an injection every six months.

• Teriparatide: An anabolic agent, teriparatide stimulates bone formation and is often prescribed for severe osteoporosis.

B. Lifestyle Modifications:

1. Importance of Weight-Bearing Exercises: Weight-bearing exercises, such as walking, jogging, and resistance training, are integral to osteoporosis management. These activities stimulate bone formation, enhance muscle strength, and improve balance, reducing the risk of falls and fractures.

2. Role of Physical Therapy: Physical therapy is valuable for individuals with osteoporosis, providing tailored exercises to improve flexibility, balance, and posture. Physical therapists work collaboratively with individuals to enhance overall musculoskeletal function, reducing the risk of falls and fractures.

3. Fall Prevention Strategies: Fall prevention is a cornerstone of osteoporosis management. Home safety assessments, addressing environmental hazards, and implementing strategies to improve balance and

coordination contribute to minimizing the risk of falls. Assistive devices, such as handrails and proper lighting, are essential components of fall prevention.

C. Nutritional Interventions:

1. Calcium and Its Role in Bone Health: Adequate calcium intake is crucial for maintaining bone density. Dietary sources of calcium include dairy products, leafy green vegetables, and fortified foods. Calcium supplements may be recommended, especially if dietary intake is insufficient. However, it's crucial to balance supplementation with considerations for overall health.

2. Vitamin D Supplementation: Vitamin D is essential for calcium absorption and bone health. Sunlight exposure, dietary sources like fatty fish and fortified foods, and vitamin D supplements contribute to maintaining optimal vitamin D levels. Healthcare professionals often assess vitamin D status and recommend supplementation as needed.

3. Protein Intake and Muscle-Bone Interactions: Protein is vital for muscle and bone health. Ensuring an adequate protein intake supports overall musculoskeletal function, contributing to bone strength and reducing the risk of fractures. Sources of lean protein, including poultry, fish, beans, and dairy, should be incorporated into the diet.

CHAPTER TWO

A well-balanced and nutrient-rich diet plays a pivotal role in supporting bone health and mitigating the risk of osteoporosis. Essential nutrients such as Calcium, vitamin D, protein, and phosphorus, along with mindful choices regarding sodium, caffeine, and alcohol intake, contribute to maintaining optimal bone density. Here, we explore the critical components of an osteoporosis-friendly diet.

A. Calcium-Rich Foods:

Dairy Products and Alternatives:

• Overview: Dairy products are excellent sources of Calcium. Opt for low-fat or non-fat milk, yoghurt, and cheese varieties to ensure adequate calcium intake without excess saturated fat.

• Impact: The body readily absorbs Calcium in dairy products, supporting bone mineralization and density.

Non-dairy sources like Leafy Greens, Nuts, and Seeds:

• Overview: Leafy green vegetables (such as kale, broccoli, and bok choy) and nuts and seeds (like almonds and chia seeds) offer alternative sources of Calcium for individuals who may be lactose intolerant or follow a plant-based diet.

• Impact: Incorporating a variety of non-dairy calcium-rich foods ensures diverse nutrient intake and supports those with dietary restrictions.

B. Vitamin D Sources:

Sun Exposure:

• Overview: Sunlight is a natural source of vitamin D. Spending time outdoors, especially during peak sunlight hours, stimulates the skin's production of vitamin D.

• Impact: Adequate sun exposure is crucial for maintaining optimal vitamin D levels, essential for calcium absorption and bone health.

Dietary Sources such as Fatty Fish and Fortified Foods:

• Overview: Fatty fish (such as salmon and mackerel) and fortified foods (like fortified milk and breakfast cereals) are dietary sources of vitamin D.

• Impact: Including these foods in the diet helps supplement vitamin D intake, especially for individuals with limited sun exposure.

C. Importance of a Well-Balanced Diet:

Protein and Its Role in Bone and Muscle Health:

• Overview: Protein is essential for bone and muscle health. The diet includes lean protein sources such as poultry, fish, beans, and tofu.

• Impact: Adequate protein intake supports bone density and muscle strength, contributing to overall skeletal health.

Phosphorus-Rich Foods:

• Overview: Phosphorus is another mineral crucial for bone health. Foods rich in phosphorus include dairy products, meat, nuts, and whole grains.

• Impact: Balancing Calcium and phosphorus intake is essential for maintaining bone mineralization and strength.

D. Limiting Sodium and Caffeine Intake:

• Overview: Excessive sodium intake can lead to calcium loss through urine. Limit processed foods and choose low-sodium alternatives. High caffeine intake may also interfere with calcium absorption.

• Impact: Moderating sodium and caffeine helps maintain a favourable calcium balance in the body, supporting bone health.

E. Moderating Alcohol Consumption:

• Overview: Excessive alcohol consumption can negatively impact bone health. Limit alcohol intake to moderate levels.

• Impact: Moderation reduces the risk of bone loss and fractures associated with heavy alcohol consumption.

F. Hydration and Its Impact on Bone Health:

• Overview: Staying hydrated is essential for overall health, including bone health. Water is a critical component of bone tissue.

• Impact: Proper hydration supports the transport of nutrients to cells, including those involved in bone formation and maintenance.

PREVENTION STRATEGIES FOR OSTEOPOROSIS

Osteoporosis, a condition characterized by weakened bones and increased susceptibility to fractures, is a largely preventable and manageable condition. Prevention strategies encompass a range of lifestyle modifications, early detection measures, and educational initiatives. Here, we explore comprehensive approaches to prevent osteoporosis and promote skeletal health.

A. Lifestyle Modifications for Prevention:

Exercise Routines:

• Overview: Regular physical activity, particularly weight-bearing and resistance exercises, is fundamental for preventing osteoporosis. Activities like walking, jogging, weightlifting, and dancing stimulate bone formation and enhance bone density.

• Impact: Exercise strengthens bones and improves balance and coordination, reducing the risk of falls and fractures.

Healthy Dietary Habits:

• Overview: Adopting a nutrient-rich and well-balanced

diet is crucial for preventing osteoporosis. Ensure adequate intake of Calcium, vitamin D, protein, and other essential nutrients through a variety of foods.

• Impact: A diet rich in bone-boosting nutrients supports optimal bone density and contributes to overall musculoskeletal health.

B. Screening and Early Detection:

Importance of Regular Check-Ups:

• Overview: Regular health check-ups, especially as individuals age, provide early detection and intervention opportunities. Healthcare professionals can assess risk factors, evaluate bone health, and provide personalized recommendations.

• Impact: Early detection allows for the timely implementation of preventive measures, reducing the risk of osteoporosis-related complications.

DXA Scans and Other Diagnostic Tools:

• Overview: Dual-energy X-ray absorptiometry (DXA) scans are the gold standard for assessing bone density. These scans measure bone mineral density at specific sites, helping identify osteoporosis and its precursor, osteopenia.

• Impact: DXA scans, along with other diagnostic tools, provide valuable information for risk stratification, guiding healthcare professionals in tailoring preventive strategies and interventions.

C. Education and Awareness Campaigns:

• Overview: Public education and awareness campaigns play a crucial role in preventing osteoporosis. These campaigns aim to inform individuals about risk factors, lifestyle choices, and the importance of early detection.

• Impact: Increased awareness empowers individuals to make informed decisions about their bone health. Education campaigns also promote the adoption of preventive measures, such as regular exercise, a balanced diet, and health check-ups.

SAMPLE MEAL PLAN

Here's a varied meal plan for seven days, focusing on supporting bone health:

DAY 1:

Breakfast:

• Greek yoghurt parfait with mixed berries (blueberries, strawberries, and raspberries)

• Granola (fortified with calcium and vitamin D)

• Almond slices for added protein and healthy fats

Lunch:

• Grilled salmon salad with mixed greens, cherry tomatoes, and avocado

• Quinoa as a side for additional protein and phosphorus

• Fresh orange slices for vitamin C, which aids calcium absorption

Snack:

• Cottage cheese with sliced peaches

• Whole grain crackers for added fibre

Dinner:

• Baked chicken breast with a side of steamed broccoli and sweet potatoes

• Brown rice for fibre and additional nutrients

• Spinach salad with feta cheese and a light vinaigrette dressing

DAY 2:

Breakfast:

• Spinach and feta omelette

• Whole grain toast with avocado

• Orange juice (fortified with vitamin D)

Lunch:

• Lentil soup with kale and tomatoes

• Whole wheat roll on the side

• Greek salad with olives and cucumber

Snack:

• Apple slices with almond butter

• Low-fat cheese cubes for calcium

Dinner:

• Grilled shrimp with asparagus and quinoa

• Roasted Brussels sprouts with a sprinkle of Parmesan cheese

• Mixed berries for dessert

DAY 3:

Breakfast:

• Smoothie with spinach, banana, almond milk, and a scoop of protein powder

• Whole grain toast with peanut butter

Lunch:

• Turkey and avocado wrap with whole wheat tortilla

• Side of carrot and celery sticks

• Hummus for dipping

Snack:

• Yogurt parfait with granola and kiwi slices

• Handful of walnuts for added omega-3 fatty acids

Dinner:

• Baked cod with a lemon and herb marinade

• Quinoa pilaf with mixed vegetables

• Steamed green beans

DAY 4:

Breakfast:

• Oatmeal topped with sliced bananas and chopped almonds

• A glass of fortified orange juice

Lunch:

• Chickpea salad with cherry tomatoes, cucumber, and feta cheese

• Whole grain pita on the side

Snack:

• Cottage cheese with pineapple chunks

• Whole grain crackers

Dinner:

• Beef stir-fry with broccoli, bell peppers, and snap peas

• Brown rice as a base

• Mixed fruit salad for dessert

DAY 5:

Breakfast:

• Whole grain pancakes with sliced strawberries and a drizzle of honey

• Scrambled eggs with spinach and feta

• A glass of fortified milk

Lunch:

• Quinoa salad with cherry tomatoes, black beans, corn, and a lime vinaigrette

• Grilled chicken breast strips

• Whole grain roll on the side

Snack:

• Greek yoghurt with a sprinkle of chia seeds

• Handful of almonds

Dinner:

• Baked tilapia with a lemon and herb crust

• Sweet potato wedges

• Steamed asparagus

DAY 6:

Breakfast:

- Smoothie bowl with mixed berries, banana slices, and a dollop of Greek yoghurt

- Whole grain toast with avocado

Lunch:

- Lentil and vegetable stew

- Quinoa and kale salad with a light balsamic dressing

- Sliced orange for dessert

Snack:

- Cottage cheese with sliced mango

- Whole grain crackers with hummus

Dinner:

- Turkey meatballs with whole-wheat spaghetti

- Tomato and spinach sauce

- Broccoli and cauliflower on the side

DAY 7:

Breakfast:

• Overnight oats with almond milk, chia seeds, and diced peaches

• Hard-boiled egg on the side

Lunch:

• Spinach and strawberry salad with grilled chicken

• Quinoa tabbouleh

• Whole grain pita bread

Snack:

• Banana smoothie with yoghurt and a scoop of protein powder

• Handful of walnuts

Dinner:

• Baked tofu with a sesame ginger glaze

• Brown rice and vegetable stir-fry

• Steamed edamame

CHAPTER THREE

Calcium-Rich Foods Recipes

Greek Yogurt Parfait with Mixed Berries and Almonds

Description: This delightful Greek Yogurt Parfait perfectly combines creamy yoghurt, vibrant mixed berries, and crunchy almonds. Packed with calcium, protein, and antioxidants, it's a wholesome and satisfying breakfast or snack option. The burst of flavours and textures makes this parfait a delicious treat that contributes to your bone health.

Ingredients:

• 1 cup non-fat Greek yogurt

• 1/2 cup mixed berries (strawberries, blueberries, raspberries)

• Two tablespoons sliced almonds

• One teaspoon of honey (optional for sweetness)

• Fresh mint leaves for garnish (optional)

Instructions:

Prepare the Greek Yogurt:

• Spoon the non-fat Greek yoghurt into a serving glass or bowl.

Add Mixed Berries:

• Wash and prepare the mixed berries. Layer them on top of the Greek yoghurt.

Sprinkle Almonds:

• Sprinkle the sliced almonds over the berries, adding a delightful crunch and a boost of healthy fats.

Drizzle with Honey (Optional):

• If you prefer a touch of sweetness, drizzle the honey over the parfait. Adjust the quantity based on your taste preference.

Garnish with Mint Leaves (Optional):

• Garnish the parfait with a few fresh mint leaves for a new and aromatic touch.

Serve and Enjoy:

• Serve the Greek Yogurt Parfait immediately, savouring the combination of creamy yoghurt, juicy berries, and crunchy almonds.

Nutrition Information (Per Serving):

• Calories: Approximately 200-220 calories

• Protein: 15g

• Carbohydrates: 25g

• Dietary Fiber: 5g

• Sugars: 15g

• Fat: 8g

• Saturated Fat: 1g

• Cholesterol: 10mg

• Sodium: 50mg

KALE AND QUINOA STUFFED PEPPERS

Description: These Kale and Quinoa Stuffed Peppers are a nutritious and satisfying meal that combines the earthy flavours of kale and quinoa with the sweetness of bell peppers. This dish is a delightful addition to your menu, packed with protein, fibre, and essential vitamins. Whether served as a main course or a vibrant side, these stuffed peppers offer a colourful and flavorful experience.

Ingredients:

- Four large bell peppers (any colour)
- 1 cup quinoa, cooked according to package instructions
- 2 cups kale, finely chopped
- One can (15 oz) black beans, drained and rinsed
- 1 cup cherry tomatoes, diced
- 1/2 cup red onion, finely chopped
- Two cloves garlic, minced
- One teaspoon cumin
- One teaspoon of chilli powder
- Salt and pepper to taste
- 1 cup shredded cheese (cheddar or Mexican blend)

- Fresh cilantro for garnish (optional)

- Lime wedges for serving

Instructions:

Preheat the Oven:

Preheat the oven to 375°F (190°C).

Prepare the Bell Peppers:

Cut the tops off the bell peppers and remove the seeds and membranes. Lightly brush the exterior of the peppers with olive oil and place them in a baking dish.

Prepare the Filling:

Combine the cooked quinoa, chopped kale, black beans, diced tomatoes, red onion, minced garlic, cumin, chilli powder, salt, and pepper in a large mixing bowl. Mix well until all ingredients are evenly incorporated.

Stuff the Peppers:

Spoon the quinoa and kale mixture into each bell pepper, pressing down gently to pack the filling.

Top with Cheese:

Sprinkle shredded cheese over the top of each stuffed pepper, covering the filling.

Bake in the Oven:

Cover the baking dish with foil and bake in the preheated oven for 25-30 minutes or until the peppers are tender.

Garnish and Serve:

Remove from the oven and garnish with fresh

cilantro if desired. Serve the stuffed peppers with lime wedges on the side for a burst of citrus flavour.

Nutrition Information (Per Serving):

• Calories: Approximately 300-350 calories

• Protein: 15g

• Carbohydrates: 45g

• Dietary Fiber: 12g

• Sugars: 5g

• Fat: 8g

• Saturated Fat: 3g

• Cholesterol: 15mg

• Sodium: 400mg

CREAMY BROCCOLI AND CHEDDAR SOUP

Description: Indulge in comfort and warmth with this velvety Creamy Broccoli and Cheddar Soup. Packed with soup is a delightful blend of flavours and textures, filled with some broccoli florets and the rich, savoury goodness of sharp cheddar cheese; this hearty soup is sure to become a family favourite, perfect for a cosy lunch or dinner.

Ingredients:

• Two tablespoons unsalted butter

• One onion, diced

• Two cloves garlic, minced

• 3 cups broccoli florets

• 3 cups low-sodium vegetable or chicken broth

• 1 cup milk (whole or 2%)

• 1/2 cup heavy cream

• 2 cups sharp cheddar cheese, shredded

• 1/4 cup all-purpose flour

• Salt and pepper to taste

• Optional toppings: additional shredded cheddar, croutons, or chopped chives

Instructions:

Sauté Aromatics:

In a large pot, melt the butter over medium heat. Add diced onions and minced garlic, sautéing until softened and fragrant.

Add Broccoli:

Incorporate the broccoli florets into the pot and cook for an additional 3-4 minutes, allowing them to soften slightly.

Prepare Roux:

Sprinkle flour over the vegetables and stir continuously to create a roux, cooking for 2-3 minutes until lightly golden.

Pour in Broth and Milk:

Gradually pour in the vegetable or chicken broth and milk, stirring constantly to avoid lumps. Bring the mixture to a gentle simmer.

Simmer and Blend:

Allow the soup to simmer for 15-20 minutes until the broccoli is tender. Use an immersion blender to puree the soup to your desired consistency. Alternatively, transfer the soup in batches to a blender, blend, and return to the pot.

Add Cheese and Cream:

Stir in the shredded cheddar cheese until thoroughly melted. Pour in the heavy cream, stirring to combine. Season with salt and pepper to taste.

Serve Hot:

Ladle the creamy soup into bowls. Top with additional shredded cheddar, croutons, or chopped chives if desired.

Enjoy:

Serve the Creamy Broccoli and Cheddar Soup hot, savouring the comforting blend of broccoli and cheesy goodness.

Nutrition Information (Per Serving):

• Calories: Approximately 300-350 calories

• Protein: 15g

• Carbohydrates: 15g

• Dietary Fiber: 3g

• Sugars: 5g

• Fat: 20g

• Saturated Fat: 12g

• Cholesterol: 60mg

• Sodium: 400mg

SARDINE AND SPINACH OMELETTE

Description: Elevate your breakfast with this protein-packed and flavorful Sardine and Spinach Omelette. Packed with omega-3 fatty acids from sardines and the nutritional goodness of spinach, this omelette is a quick, nutritious, and delicious way to start your day. The combination of savoury sardines and vibrant spinach creates a delightful harmony of flavours that will satisfy your taste buds and provide a nutrient boost.

Ingredients:

• Three large eggs

• One can (4.375 oz) sardines in olive oil, drained

• 1 cup fresh spinach leaves, chopped

• 1/4 cup red bell pepper, diced

• 1/4 cup feta cheese, crumbled

• One tablespoon of olive oil

• Salt and pepper to taste

• Fresh parsley for garnish (optional)

Instructions:

Prepare the Sardines:

Drain the sardines from the olive oil. If desired, break the sardines into smaller pieces.

Whisk the Eggs:

In a bowl, whisk the eggs until well combined. Season with salt and pepper according to your taste.

Sauté Vegetables:

Heat olive oil in a non-stick skillet over medium heat. Add diced red bell pepper and chopped spinach, sautéing until the spinach wilts and the bell pepper softens.

Add Sardines:

Add the drained sardines to the skillet, distributing them evenly among the vegetables.

Pour in Whisked Eggs:

Pour the whisked eggs over the sardines and vegetables, ensuring an even distribution.

Cook and Fold:

Allow the eggs to set around the edges. Gently lift the edges with a spatula, allowing the uncooked eggs to flow underneath. Once the omelette is mostly set but still slightly runny on top, fold it in half.

Add Feta Cheese:

Sprinkle crumbled feta cheese over one-half of the omelette. Fold the other half over the cheese, creating a half-moon shape.

Finish Cooking:

Continue cooking for another minute or until the cheese melts and the omelette is cooked to your desired level of doneness.

Garnish and Serve:

Slide the Sardine and Spinach Omelette onto a plate. Garnish with fresh parsley if desired.

Enjoy:

Serve the omelette hot, savouring the delicious combination of sardines, spinach, and feta.

Nutrition Information (Per Serving):

• Calories: Approximately 350-400 calories

• Protein: 25g

• Carbohydrates: 4g

• Dietary Fiber: 1g

• Sugars: 1g

• Fat: 28g

• Saturated Fat: 7g

• Cholesterol: 535mg

• Sodium: 550mg

BAKED SWEET POTATO WITH GREEK YOGURT AND POMEGRANATE SEEDS

Description: Satisfy your taste buds and nourish your body with this delectable, nutrient-packed Baked Sweet Potato topped with creamy Greek yoghurt and vibrant pomegranate seeds. Bursting with flavours and textures, this dish combines the natural sweetness of baked sweet potatoes with the tangy richness of Greek yoghurt and the juicy pop of pomegranate seeds. It's a delightful and visually appealing treat that makes for a wholesome snack or a unique side dish.

Ingredients:

- Two medium-sized sweet potatoes
- 1 cup Greek yogurt (unsweetened)
- 1/2 cup pomegranate seeds

· One tablespoon honey (optional for drizzling)

· One tablespoon chopped fresh mint leaves (optional for garnish)

Instructions:

Preheat the Oven:

Preheat your oven to 400°F (200°C).

Prepare the Sweet Potatoes:

Scrub the sweet potatoes thoroughly and pierce them with a fork in several places. Place them on a baking sheet lined with parchment paper.

Bake the Sweet Potatoes:

Bake the sweet potatoes in the preheated oven for 45-60 minutes or until they are tender and can be easily pierced with a fork.

Slice and Fluff:

Once baked, slice each sweet potato open lengthwise. Gently fluff the insides with a fork to create a fluffy texture.

Add Greek Yogurt:

Spoon a generous dollop of Greek yoghurt onto each sweet potato half, spreading it evenly.

Sprinkle Pomegranate Seeds:

Sprinkle a generous amount of fresh pomegranate seeds over the Greek yoghurt, creating a colourful and juicy topping.

Drizzle with Honey (Optional):

For added sweetness, drizzle honey over the sweet potatoes. Adjust the quantity based on your taste preference.

Garnish with Mint (Optional):

Garnish the dish with chopped fresh mint leaves for a burst of freshness.

Serve and Enjoy:

Serve the Baked Sweet Potato with Greek Yogurt and Pomegranate Seeds immediately, relishing the combination of creamy, sweet, and tart flavours.

Nutrition Information (Per Serving):

• Calories: Approximately 200-250 calories

• Protein: 10g

• Carbohydrates: 40g

• Dietary Fiber: 7g

• Sugars: 15g

• Fat: 2g

• Saturated Fat: 1g

• Cholesterol: 10mg

• Sodium: 60mg

TOFU AND VEGETABLE STIR-FRY

Description: Experience a burst of flavours and textures with this Tofu and Vegetable Stir-Fry—a vibrant and wholesome dish that combines the protein-packed goodness of tofu with an array of colourful vegetables. Stir-frying ensures that each bite is infused with savoury sauces, creating a delicious and nutritious meal that's quick to prepare. Whether served over rice or noodles, this stir-fry perfectly balances freshness and satisfying heartiness.

Ingredients:

- One block (14 oz) of firm tofu, pressed and cubed

- Two tablespoons soy sauce (low-sodium)

- One tablespoon of hoisin sauce

- One tablespoon of sesame oil

- One tablespoon cornstarch

- Two tablespoons vegetable oil (for stir-frying)

- 1 cup broccoli florets

- One bell pepper (any colour), thinly sliced

- One carrot, julienned

- 1 cup snap peas, ends trimmed

- Three green onions, sliced

- Two cloves garlic, minced

- One teaspoon of fresh ginger, grated

- Sesame seeds for garnish (optional)

- Cooked brown rice or noodles for serving

Instructions:

Prepare Tofu:

Press the tofu to remove excess water. Cut it into cubes and toss it with one tablespoon of soy sauce, hoisin sauce, sesame oil, and cornstarch. Allow it to marinate for at least 15 minutes.

Stir-Fry Tofu:

Heat one tablespoon of vegetable oil in a wok or large skillet over medium-high heat. Add the marinated tofu and stir-fry until golden brown on all sides. Remove the tofu from the pan and set aside.

Stir-Fry Vegetables:

In the same pan, add another tablespoon of vegetable oil. Stir-fry the broccoli, bell pepper, carrot, and snap peas until they are tender-crisp.

Add Aromatics:

Add minced garlic and grated ginger to the vegetables, stirring for about 30 seconds until fragrant.

Combine Tofu and Vegetables:

Return the cooked tofu to the pan with the vegetables, tossing everything together to combine.

Season with Soy Sauce:

Drizzle the remaining soy sauce over the tofu and vegetables, ensuring an even distribution. Adjust seasoning to taste.

Finish and Garnish:

Add sliced green onions and sesame seeds for garnish. Toss briefly to incorporate.

Serve:

Serve the Tofu and Vegetable Stir-Fry over cooked brown rice or noodles, enjoying the delightful mix of textures and flavours.

Nutrition Information (Per Serving, without rice/noodles):

• Calories: Approximately 300-350 calories

• Protein: 20g

• Carbohydrates: 20g

• Dietary Fiber: 6g

• Sugars: 6g

• Fat: 18g

• Saturated Fat: 2g

• Cholesterol: 0mg

• Sodium: 700mg

MANGO AND KALE SMOOTHIE WITH CHIA SEEDS

Description: Indulge in a refreshing and nutrient-packed treat with this Mango and Kale Smoothie featuring the added goodness of chia seeds. This vibrant and green smoothie is a delicious way to incorporate the powerhouse nutrients of kale, the tropical sweetness of mango, and the omega-3 fatty acids from chia seeds. Start your day with a burst of energy and a dose of essential vitamins with this wholesome and satisfying smoothie.

Ingredients:

• 1 cup fresh kale leaves, stems removed

• 1 cup frozen mango chunks

• 1/2 banana

• One tablespoon of chia seeds

• 1 cup unsweetened almond milk (or any milk of choice)

• 1/2 cup Greek yoghurt (optional for creaminess)

• Ice cubes (optional)

• Honey or agave syrup for sweetness (optional)

Instructions:

Prepare Ingredients:

Wash the kale leaves thoroughly and remove the stems. Cut or tear them into smaller pieces for more effortless blending.

Combine in Blender:

Combine the kale leaves, frozen mango chunks, banana, chia seeds, almond milk, and Greek yoghurt (if using). Add ice cubes if a colder consistency is desired.

Blend Until Smooth:

Blend the ingredients on high speed until the smoothie reaches a creamy and smooth consistency.

Adjust Sweetness (Optional):

Taste the smoothie and, if desired, add honey or agave syrup to sweeten according to your preference. Blend again to incorporate.

Serve:

Pour the Mango and Kale Smoothie into a glass. Sprinkle additional chia seeds on top for added texture if desired.

Enjoy Immediately:

Sip and enjoy the refreshing and nutritious goodness of this Mango and Kale Smoothie with Chia Seeds.

Nutrition Information (Approximate):

• Calories: Approximately 250-300 calories

• Protein: 8g

- Carbohydrates: 45g
- Dietary Fiber: 10g
- Sugars: 25g
- Fat: 8g
- Saturated Fat: 1g
- Cholesterol: 5mg
- Sodium: 150mg

CHEESE AND SPINACH STUFFED CHICKEN BREAST

Description: Elevate your dinner with this indulgent yet easy-to-make Cheese and Spinach Stuffed Chicken Breast. Juicy chicken breasts are filled with a flavorful mixture of creamy cheese and nutrient-packed spinach, creating a delicious and visually appealing dish. Whether served as a centrepiece for a special occasion or a delightful family meal, this stuffed chicken breast is sure to impress with its lovely combination of textures and tastes.

Ingredients:

• Four boneless, skinless chicken breasts

• 1 cup fresh spinach, chopped

• 1 cup shredded mozzarella cheese

• 1/2 cup feta cheese, crumbled

• Two cloves garlic, minced

• One teaspoon dried oregano

• Salt and pepper to taste

• Olive oil for drizzling

• Toothpicks or kitchen twine for securing

Instructions:

Preheat the Oven:

Preheat your oven to 375°F (190°C).

Prepare Chicken Breasts:

Lay each chicken breast flat on a cutting board. With a sharp knife, make a horizontal slit along the side of each chicken breast to create a pocket. Be careful not to cut through the other side.

Season Chicken:

Season the inside of each chicken breast with salt, pepper, and dried oregano.

Make the Filling:

In a bowl, combine chopped spinach, mozzarella cheese, feta cheese, minced garlic, salt, and pepper. Mix well.

Stuff the Chicken:

Spoon the cheese and spinach mixture into the pockets of the chicken breasts, pressing down gently to ensure they are well-filled.

Secure with Toothpicks or Twine:

If using toothpicks, secure the open end of the chicken breast with toothpicks to keep the stuffing inside. If using kitchen twine, tie the chicken breasts securely.

Drizzle with Olive Oil:

Place the stuffed chicken breasts on a baking sheet. Drizzle olive oil over the top of each breast for a golden finish.

Bake in the Oven:

Bake in the preheated oven for 25-30 minutes or until the chicken is cooked, with an internal temperature of 165°F (74°C).

Rest and Slice:

Allow the stuffed chicken breasts to rest for a few minutes before slicing. Remove toothpicks or twine before serving.

Serve:

Serve the Cheese and Spinach Stuffed Chicken Breast with your favourite sides, such as roasted vegetables, quinoa, or a fresh salad.

Nutrition Information (Per Serving):

• Calories: Approximately 300-350 calories

• Protein: 40g

• Carbohydrates: 3g

• Dietary Fiber: 1g

• Sugars: 1g

• Fat: 16g

• Saturated Fat: 8g

• Cholesterol: 120mg

• Sodium: 500mg

CHAPTER FOUR

Protein-Rich Foods Recipes

Grilled Chicken Quinoa Bowl with Avocado

Description: Enjoy a wholesome and satisfying meal with this Grilled Chicken Quinoa Bowl featuring the creamy richness of avocado. Packed with protein, fibre, and a variety of textures, this bowl is a delightful combination of grilled chicken, nutrient-rich quinoa, and the buttery goodness of ripe avocado. Whether enjoyed for lunch or dinner, this bowl is a perfect balance of flavours and nutrition.

Ingredients:

For the Grilled Chicken:

• Two boneless, skinless chicken breasts

• One tablespoon of olive oil

• One teaspoon of smoked paprika

• One teaspoon of garlic powder

• Salt and pepper to taste

• Fresh lemon wedges for serving

For the Quinoa:

• 1 cup quinoa, rinsed

• 2 cups water or chicken broth

• Salt to taste

For the Bowl:

• One ripe avocado, sliced

• 1 cup cherry tomatoes, halved

• One cucumber, diced

- 1/4 cup red onion, finely chopped
- Fresh cilantro or parsley for garnish
- Lemon or lime wedges for extra citrus flavour

Instructions:

Preheat Grill:

Preheat your grill to medium-high heat.

Season Chicken:

Combine olive oil, smoked paprika, garlic powder, salt, and pepper in a bowl. Rub the mixture evenly over the chicken breasts.

Grill Chicken:

Grill the chicken breasts for 6-8 minutes per side or until fully cooked with an internal temperature of 165°F (74°C). Remove from the grill and let them rest for a few minutes before slicing.

Prepare Quinoa:

Combine quinoa, water or broth, and a pinch of salt in a saucepan. Bring to a boil, then reduce the heat to low, cover, and simmer for 15-20 minutes or until the quinoa is cooked and the liquid is absorbed.

Assemble the Bowl:

In individual serving bowls, layer cooked quinoa, sliced grilled chicken, avocado slices, cherry tomatoes, diced cucumber, and finely chopped red onion.

Garnish:

Garnish the bowl with fresh cilantro or parsley.

Add a squeeze of lemon or lime juice for extra freshness.

Serve:

Serve the Grilled Chicken Quinoa Bowl with Avocado immediately, savouring the combination of grilled flavours, creamy avocado, and vibrant vegetables.

Nutrition Information (Per Serving):

• Calories: Approximately 400-450 calories

• Protein: 30g

• Carbohydrates: 40g

• Dietary Fiber: 8g

• Sugars: 3g

• Fat: 16g

• Saturated Fat: 2g

• Cholesterol: 60mg

• Sodium: 300mg

BLACK BEAN AND VEGETABLE CHILI

Description: Indulge in a guilt-free and delicious meal with this Light and Flavorful Black Bean and Vegetable Chili. Packed with vibrant vegetables, protein-rich black beans, and a blend of savoury spices, this chilli is a satisfying dish that won't weigh you down. Each spoonful is a celebration of wholesome ingredients and bold flavours, making it an ideal choice for a nourishing dinner.

Ingredients:

• Two tablespoons of olive oil

• One large onion, diced

• Three cloves garlic, minced

• One bell pepper (any colour), diced

• One zucchini, diced

• One carrot, diced

• 1 cup corn kernels (fresh, frozen, or canned)

• Two cans (15 oz each) of black beans, drained and rinsed

• One can (28 oz) crushed tomatoes

• 1 cup vegetable broth

• Two tablespoons of chilli powder

- One tablespoon cumin

- One teaspoon paprika

- 1/2 teaspoon cayenne pepper (optional for heat)

- Salt and pepper to taste

- Fresh cilantro or green onions for garnish

- Optional toppings: shredded cheese, sour cream, avocado slices

Instructions:

Sauté Vegetables:

In a large pot, heat olive oil over medium heat. Add diced onion, minced garlic, bell pepper, zucchini, and carrot. Sauté until the vegetables are softened, about 5-7 minutes.

Add Beans and Corn:

Stir in black beans and corn, combining them well with the sautéed vegetables.

Season the Chili:

Sprinkle chilli powder, cumin, paprika, cayenne pepper (if using), salt, and pepper over the vegetable mixture. Stir well to coat the vegetables and beans with the spices.

Pour in Tomatoes and Broth:

Add crushed tomatoes and vegetable broth to the pot. Stir to combine.

Simmer:

Bring the chilli to a simmer. Reduce the heat to low, cover, and let it simmer for at least 20-30 minutes to allow the flavours to meld. Stir occasionally.

Adjust Seasoning:

Taste the chilli and adjust the seasoning as needed. Add more salt, pepper, or spices according to your preference.

Serve:

Ladle the Black Bean and Vegetable Chili into bowls. Garnish with fresh cilantro or green onions, and add optional toppings like shredded cheese, sour cream, or avocado slices.

Enjoy:

Serve the chilli hot, savouring the rich flavours and comforting warmth.

Nutrition Information (Per Serving):

• Calories: Approximately 220 calories

• Protein: 10g

• Carbohydrates: 35g

• Dietary Fiber: 10g

• Sugars: 8g

• Fat: 6g

• Saturated Fat: 1g

• Cholesterol: 0mg

• Sodium: 400mg

TURKEY AND QUINOA STUFFED BELL PEPPERS

Description: Delight your taste buds with these wholesome, protein-packed Turkey and Quinoa Stuffed Bell Peppers. This nutritious and flavorful dish combines lean ground turkey, hearty quinoa, and a medley of vegetables, creating a satisfying meal as delicious as nourishing. Perfect for a well-balanced dinner, these stuffed bell peppers are a colourful and tasty addition to your repertoire of healthy recipes.

Ingredients:

For the Stuffed Bell Peppers:

- Four large bell peppers (any colour)

- 1 cup quinoa, cooked according to package instructions

- 1 lb lean ground turkey

- One onion, finely chopped

- Two cloves garlic, minced

- 1 cup cherry tomatoes, diced

- 1 cup black beans, drained and rinsed

- 1 cup corn kernels (fresh, frozen, or canned)

- One teaspoon of ground cumin

- One teaspoon of chili powder

- Salt and pepper to taste

- 1 cup shredded cheese (cheddar, Monterey Jack, or your choice)

- Fresh cilantro or parsley for garnish

For the Tomato Sauce:

- One can (14 oz) crushed tomatoes

- One teaspoon dried oregano

- 1/2 teaspoon garlic powder

- Salt and pepper to taste

Instructions:

Preheat the Oven:

Preheat your oven to 375°F (190°C).

Prepare Bell Peppers:

Cut the tops off the bell peppers and remove the seeds and membranes. If needed, slice a small portion off the bottom to help them stand upright in the baking dish.

Cook Quinoa:

Cook quinoa according to package instructions. Set aside.

Prepare Turkey Mixture:

In a large skillet, cook ground turkey over medium heat until browned. Add chopped onions and minced garlic, sautéing until the onions are translucent.

Add Vegetables and Quinoa:

Stir in diced cherry tomatoes, black beans, corn, cooked quinoa, ground cumin, chilli powder, salt, and pepper. Mix well to combine.

Make Tomato Sauce:

Mix crushed tomatoes with dried oregano, garlic powder, salt, and pepper in a separate bowl. Set aside.

Stuff Bell Peppers:

Stuff each bell pepper with the turkey and quinoa mixture. Place the stuffed peppers in a baking dish.

Pour Tomato Sauce:

Pour the tomato sauce over the stuffed peppers, ensuring they are well covered.

Bake:

Cover the baking dish with aluminium foil and bake in the preheated oven for 25-30 minutes or until the peppers are tender.

Add Cheese and Garnish:

Remove the foil, sprinkle shredded cheese over each stuffed pepper, and return to the oven until the cheese is melted and bubbly.

Serve:

Garnish with fresh cilantro or parsley. Serve the hot Turkey and Quinoa Stuffed Bell Peppers and enjoy a wholesome, well-balanced meal.

Nutrition Information (Per Serving):

• Calories: Approximately 300-350 calories

- Protein: 25g
- Carbohydrates: 35g
- Dietary Fiber: 8g
- Sugars: 6g
- Fat: 10g
- Saturated Fat: 4g
- Cholesterol: 60mg
- Sodium: 500mg

LENTIL AND CHICKPEA SALAD WITH FETA

Description: Savor the wholesome goodness of this Lentil and Chickpea Salad with Feta—a vibrant and protein-packed dish that combines the earthy flavours of lentils and chickpeas with the creamy richness of feta cheese. Bursting with fresh vegetables and tossed in a zesty vinaigrette, this salad is a delightful addition to your repertoire of nutritious and satisfying meals. Enjoy it as a light lunch, a refreshing side, or a standalone dish that celebrates the harmony of textures and tastes.

Ingredients:

For the Salad:

- 1 cup green or brown lentils, cooked and cooled

- One can (15 oz) chickpeas, drained and rinsed

- One cucumber, diced

- One bell pepper (any colour), diced

- 1 cup cherry tomatoes, halved

- 1/2 red onion, finely chopped

- 1/2 cup Kalamata olives, sliced

- 1/2 cup crumbled feta cheese
- Fresh parsley or mint for garnish

For the Vinaigrette:

- 1/4 cup extra-virgin olive oil
- Two tablespoons of red wine vinegar
- One teaspoon of Dijon mustard
- One clove of garlic, minced
- Salt and pepper to taste

Instructions:

Cook Lentils:

Cook lentils according to package instructions. Once cooked, let them cool.

Prepare Vinaigrette:

Whisk together olive oil, red wine vinegar, Dijon mustard, minced garlic, salt, and pepper in a small bowl. Set aside.

Assemble Salad:

Combine cooked lentils, chickpeas, diced cucumber, bell pepper, cherry tomatoes, chopped red onion, sliced Kalamata olives, and crumbled feta cheese in a large salad bowl.

Toss with Vinaigrette:

Drizzle the vinaigrette over the salad and gently toss to coat all ingredients evenly.

Garnish:

Garnish the Lentil and Chickpea Salad with Feta with fresh parsley or mint.

Chill (Optional):

Allow the salad to chill in the refrigerator for at least 30 minutes before serving to enhance flavours.

Serve:

Serve the salad as a refreshing and nutritious dish, celebrating the delightful combination of lentils, chickpeas, and feta.

Nutrition Information (Per Serving):

• Calories: Approximately 300-350 calories

• Protein: 15g

• Carbohydrates: 35g

• Dietary Fiber: 10g

• Sugars: 5g

• Fat: 15g

• Saturated Fat: 4g

• Cholesterol: 15mg

• Sodium: 400mg

SHRIMP AND EDAMAME STIR-FRY

Description: Embark on a culinary journey with this Shrimp and Edamame Stir-Fry—a delightful fusion of succulent shrimp, vibrant vegetables, and protein-rich edamame. Bursting with flavours and tossed in a savoury stir-fry sauce, this dish is a quick and wholesome addition to your repertoire of easy-to-make meals. Elevate your dining experience with this colourful and nutritious stir-fry that brings together the freshness of shrimp and the goodness of edamame.

Ingredients:

For the Stir-Fry:

- 1 lb large shrimp, peeled and deveined

- 2 cups edamame (fresh or frozen)

- One red bell pepper, sliced

- One yellow bell pepper, sliced

- One carrot, julienned

- 1 cup sugar snap peas, trimmed

- Three green onions, sliced

- Three cloves garlic, minced

- One tablespoon of fresh ginger, grated

- Sesame seeds for garnish (optional)
- Cooked brown rice or noodles for serving

For the Stir-Fry Sauce:

- 1/4 cup low-sodium soy sauce
- Two tablespoons of oyster sauce
- One tablespoon of honey or maple syrup
- One tablespoon of rice vinegar
- One teaspoon of sesame oil
- One teaspoon cornstarch

Instructions:

Prepare Shrimp:

Pat the shrimp dry and season with salt and pepper. Set aside.

Boil Edamame:

If using fresh edamame, boil them in salted water for 3-5 minutes. If using frozen edamame, follow package instructions. Drain and set aside.

Mix Stir-Fry Sauce:

Whisk together soy sauce, oyster sauce, honey (or maple syrup), rice vinegar, sesame oil, and cornstarch in a small bowl. Set aside.

Stir-Fry Shrimp:

Heat a large wok or skillet over medium-high heat. Add a small amount of oil and stir-fry the shrimp until they turn pink and opaque. Remove shrimp from the pan and set aside.

Sauté Vegetables:

In the same pan, add a bit more oil if needed. Sauté garlic and ginger until fragrant. Add sliced bell peppers, julienned carrot, and sugar snap peas. Stir-fry until the vegetables are crisp-tender.

Combine Shrimp, Edamame, and Sauce:

Add the cooked shrimp and boiled edamame to the pan. Pour the prepared stir-fry sauce over the mixture. Toss everything together until well-coated and heated through.

Finish and Garnish:

Stir in sliced green onions. Garnish with sesame seeds if desired.

Serve:

Serve the Shrimp and Edamame Stir-Fry over cooked brown rice or noodles, savouring the vibrant flavours and textures.

Nutrition Information (Per Serving, without rice/noodles):

• Calories: Approximately 300-350 calories

• Protein: 30g

• Carbohydrates: 20g

• Dietary Fiber: 5g

• Sugars: 8g

• Fat: 12g

• Saturated Fat: 2g

• Cholesterol: 150mg

• Sodium: 800mg

CHICKEN AND VEGETABLE SKEWERS WITH PEANUT SAUCE

Description: Elevate your grilling experience with these Chicken and Vegetable Skewers featuring a delectable Peanut Sauce. Succulent chicken pieces and colourful vegetables are threaded onto skewers, grilled to perfection, and served with a rich and savoury peanut sauce. This dish is a celebration of bold flavours, making it an ideal choice for a delightful and satisfying meal that brings a taste of Asian-inspired cuisine to your table.

Ingredients:

For the Skewers:

• 1.5 lbs boneless, skinless chicken breasts cut into chunks

• Two bell peppers (any colour), cut into chunks

• One red onion, cut into chunks

• One zucchini, sliced into rounds

• Wooden or metal skewers, soaked if wooden

For the Marinade:

- 1/4 cup soy sauce

- Two tablespoons honey

- Two tablespoons of olive oil

- Two cloves garlic, minced

- One teaspoon of ginger, grated

- One teaspoon of sesame oil

- Salt and pepper to taste

For the Peanut Sauce:

- 1/2 cup creamy peanut butter

- Three tablespoons soy sauce

- Two tablespoons of rice vinegar

- One tablespoon honey

- One clove of garlic, minced

- One teaspoon of ginger, grated

- 1/4 cup water (adjust for desired consistency)

- Crushed red pepper flakes (optional for heat)

Instructions:

Marinate Chicken:

Whisk together soy sauce, honey, olive oil, minced garlic, grated ginger, sesame oil, salt, and pepper in a bowl. Add chicken chunks to the marinade, ensuring they are well coated. Marinate for at least 30 minutes.

Prepare Peanut Sauce:

Combine peanut butter, soy sauce, rice vinegar,

honey, minced garlic, grated ginger, and water in a separate bowl. Whisk until smooth. Add crushed red pepper flakes if you like a bit of heat. Set aside.

Assemble Skewers:

Preheat the grill. Thread marinated chicken, bell peppers, red onion, and zucchini onto skewers in alternating order.

Grill Skewers:

Grill the skewers over medium-high heat, turning occasionally, until the chicken is cooked through and the vegetables are charred at the edges. This takes about 10-15 minutes.

Serve:

Arrange the Chicken and Vegetable Skewers on a platter. Drizzle the Peanut Sauce over the skewers or serve it on the side for dipping.

Garnish:

Garnish with chopped cilantro or sliced green onions.

Enjoy:

Serve immediately, savouring the grilled perfection of the Chicken and Vegetable Skewers with the irresistible Peanut Sauce.

Nutrition Information (Per Serving):

• Calories: Approximately 350-400 calories

• Protein: 30g

• Carbohydrates: 20g

• Dietary Fiber: 4g

- Sugars: 10g
- Fat: 18g
- Saturated Fat: 3g
- Cholesterol: 70mg
- Sodium: 600mg

BEEF AND BROCCOLI STIR-FRY

Description: Treat your taste buds to the savoury delights of this Beef and Broccoli Stir-Fry—an enticing blend of tender beef slices, crisp broccoli florets, and a flavorful stir-fry sauce. Quick to prepare and burst with Asian-inspired flavours, this dish is perfect for a satisfying and wholesome meal. Enjoy the irresistible combination of savoury beef, vibrant broccoli, and a mouthwatering sauce that will elevate your stir-fry experience.

Ingredients:

For the Stir-Fry:

• 1 lb flank steak, thinly sliced against the grain

• 4 cups broccoli florets

• One red bell pepper, thinly sliced

• Three cloves garlic, minced

• One tablespoon of fresh ginger, grated

• Three green onions, sliced

• Sesame seeds for garnish (optional)

• Cooked white or brown rice for serving

For the Stir-Fry Sauce:

• 1/3 cup low-sodium soy sauce

- Two tablespoons of oyster sauce
- One tablespoon of hoisin sauce
- One tablespoon cornstarch
- One tablespoon of brown sugar
- One teaspoon of sesame oil
- 1/2 cup beef broth or water

Instructions:

Prepare Stir-Fry Sauce:

Whisk together soy sauce, oyster sauce, hoisin sauce, cornstarch, brown sugar, sesame oil, and beef broth in a bowl. Set aside.

Slice Beef:

Thinly slice the flank steak against the grain. This ensures tenderness in the final dish.

Blanch Broccoli:

Blanch the broccoli florets in boiling water for 2 minutes or until slightly tender. Drain and set aside.

Stir-Fry Beef:

Heat a wok or large skillet over high heat. Add a bit of oil and stir-fry the sliced beef until browned and cooked through. Remove beef from the wok and set aside.

Sauté Aromatics:

In the same wok, add a bit more oil if needed. Sauté minced garlic and grated ginger until fragrant.

Add Vegetables:

Add sliced red bell pepper and blanched broccoli to the wok. Stir-fry for 2-3 minutes until the vegetables are crisp-tender.

Combine Beef and Sauce:

Return the cooked beef to the wok. Pour the prepared stir-fry sauce over the meat and vegetables. Toss everything together until well-coated and heated through.

Garnish and Serve:

If desired, garnish the Beef and Broccoli Stir-Fry with sliced green onions and sesame seeds. Serve over cooked rice.

Enjoy:

Dive into the delightful flavours of this Beef and Broccoli Stir-Fry, relishing the perfect balance of savoury beef and vibrant broccoli.

Nutrition Information (Per Serving, without rice):

• Calories: Approximately 350-400 calories

• Protein: 25g

• Carbohydrates: 15g

• Dietary Fiber: 4g

• Sugars: 5g

• Fat: 20g

• Saturated Fat: 6g

• Cholesterol: 60mg

• Sodium: 800mg

CHAPTER FIVE

Phosphorus-Rich Foods Recipes

Baked Potato Wedges with Garlic Aioli

Description: Satisfy your craving for a crispy and flavorful snack with these Baked Potato Wedges paired with a zesty Garlic Aioli. These wedges are seasoned to perfection, oven-baked until golden and crispy, and served with a creamy garlic-infused dipping sauce. Whether enjoyed as a delicious side dish or a tasty appetizer, these potato wedges are a crowd-pleaser that combines simplicity with irresistible flavours.

Ingredients:

For the Potato Wedges:

• Four large russet potatoes, scrubbed and cut into wedges

• Two tablespoons of olive oil

• One teaspoon of garlic powder

• One teaspoon paprika

• One teaspoon of dried thyme

• Salt and black pepper to taste

For the Garlic Aioli:

• 1/2 cup mayonnaise

• One tablespoon of Dijon mustard

• Two cloves garlic, minced

• One tablespoon of fresh lemon juice

• Salt and black pepper to taste

Instructions:

   Preheat Oven:

Preheat the oven to 425°F (220°C).

Prepare Potato Wedges:

In a large bowl, toss the potato wedges with olive oil, garlic powder, paprika, dried thyme, salt, and black pepper. Ensure the wedges are evenly coated with the seasoning.

Arrange on Baking Sheet:

Arrange the seasoned potato wedges in a single layer on a baking sheet, ensuring they are not overcrowded.

Bake:

Bake in the preheated oven for 30-35 minutes or until the wedges are golden and crispy, flipping them halfway through the baking time for even cooking.

Make Garlic Aioli:

While the potato wedges are baking, prepare the garlic aioli. Mix mayonnaise, Dijon mustard, minced garlic, fresh lemon juice, salt, and black pepper in a small bowl. Adjust the seasoning to taste.

Serve:

Once the potato wedges are golden and crispy, remove them from the oven. Serve the wedges hot with the prepared Garlic Aioli for dipping.

Garnish (Optional):

Garnish the potato wedges with fresh chopped parsley or chives for added freshness.

Enjoy:

Dive into the crispy goodness of these Baked Potato Wedges, savouring each bite dipped in the flavorful Garlic Aioli.

Note: Feel free to customize the seasoning based on your preferences. Adding a pinch of cayenne pepper or smoked paprika can add a hint of heat to the wedges.

Nutrition Information (Per Serving):

• Calories: Approximately 250-300 calories

• Carbohydrates: 30g

• Dietary Fiber: 4g

• Sugars: 2g

• Fat: 15g

• Saturated Fat: 2g

• Cholesterol: 5mg

• Sodium: 300mg

PUMPKIN SEED CRUSTED TILAPIA

Description: Experience a delightful twist on tilapia with this Pumpkin Seed pumpkin-crusted tilapia—a flavorful and nutty dish that adds a unique crunch to the tender fish fillets. The pumpkin seed crust, seasoned to perfection, creates a delicious contrast to the mild flavour of tilapia. This easy-to-make recipe is a celebration of textures and tastes, making it a perfect choice for a quick and impressive dinner.

Ingredients:

For the Pumpkin Seed Crust:

• 1 cup pumpkin seeds (pepitas), unsalted

• 1/2 cup breadcrumbs (preferably panko)

• One teaspoon of garlic powder

• One teaspoon paprika

• 1/2 teaspoon cumin

• Salt and black pepper to taste

For the Tilapia:

• Four tilapia fillets

• Two tablespoons of Dijon mustard

• One tablespoon of olive oil

• Lemon wedges for serving

Instructions:

Preheat Oven:

Preheat the oven to 400°F (200°C).

Prepare Pumpkin Seed Crust:

Combine pumpkin seeds, breadcrumbs, garlic powder, paprika, cumin, salt, and black pepper in a food processor. Pulse until the pumpkin seeds are finely ground and the mixture resembles coarse crumbs. Transfer to a shallow dish.

Coat Tilapia Fillets:

Brush each tilapia fillet with Dijon mustard, ensuring an even coating on both sides.

Crust the Tilapia:

Press each mustard-coated tilapia fillet into the pumpkin seed mixture, coating both sides generously. Gently press the crust onto the fillets to adhere.

Heat Olive Oil:

In an oven-safe skillet, heat olive oil over medium-high heat.

Sear Tilapia:

Place the pumpkin seed-crusted tilapia fillets in the hot skillet. Sear for 2-3 minutes on each side until the crust is golden brown.

Transfer to Oven:

Transfer the skillet to the preheated oven and bake for 8-10 minutes or until the tilapia is cooked through and quickly flakes with a fork.

Serve:

Remove from the oven and serve the Pumpkin Seed Crusted Tilapia hot. Squeeze lemon wedges over the fillets before serving.

Enjoy:

Enjoy the delightful combination of the nutty pumpkin seed crust and the tender tilapia, creating a memorable dining experience.

Note: This recipe works well with other white fish fillets like cod or sole. Adjust the baking time based on the thickness of the fillets.

Nutrition Information (Per Serving):

• Calories: Approximately 250-300 calories

• Protein: 30g

• Carbohydrates: 10g

• Dietary Fiber: 3g

• Sugars: 1g

• Fat: 12g

• Saturated Fat: 2g

• Cholesterol: 60mg

• Sodium: 300mg

WHOLE WHEAT PASTA WITH CHICKEN AND SUN-DRIED TOMATOES

Description: Indulge in a wholesome and flavorful meal with this Whole Wheat Pasta with Chicken and Sun-Dried Tomatoes—a hearty dish that combines the nutty goodness of whole wheat pasta with tender chicken and the intense sweetness of sun-dried tomatoes. This easy-to-make recipe is a celebration of Mediterranean-inspired flavours, creating a satisfying and nutritious dinner option for any occasion.

Ingredients:

For the Pasta:

• 8 ounces whole wheat pasta (spaghetti, penne, or your choice)

• Two boneless, skinless chicken breasts, thinly sliced

• One tablespoon of olive oil

• Three cloves garlic, minced

• 1/2 teaspoon dried oregano

- 1/2 teaspoon dried basil

- Salt and black pepper to taste

For the Sauce:

- 1/2 cup sun-dried tomatoes (not in oil), chopped

- 1 cup cherry tomatoes, halved

- 1/4 cup black olives, sliced

- 1/4 cup feta cheese, crumbled

- Two tablespoons fresh basil, chopped

- Two tablespoons pine nuts, toasted (optional)

- Red pepper flakes for a hint of heat (optional)

Instructions:

Cook Whole Wheat Pasta:

Cook the whole wheat pasta according to package instructions. Drain and set aside.

Prepare Chicken:

Season the thinly sliced chicken breasts with dried oregano, dried basil, salt, and black pepper.

Sauté Chicken:

In a large skillet, heat olive oil over medium-high heat. Add minced garlic and sauté for a minute until fragrant. Add the seasoned chicken slices and cook until browned and cooked through. Remove chicken from the skillet and set aside.

Make the Sauce:

Add sun-dried tomatoes, cherry tomatoes, black olives, and cooked chicken in the same skillet. Toss to combine and let it cook for a few minutes until the tomatoes are slightly softened.

Combine with Pasta:

Add the cooked whole wheat pasta to the skillet, tossing everything together to combine.

Add Feta and Fresh Basil:

Sprinkle crumbled feta cheese and fresh basil over the pasta. Toss gently to incorporate the cheese and basil throughout the dish.

Garnish and Serve:

If using, sprinkle toasted pine nuts over the pasta. Add red pepper flakes for a touch of heat if desired.

Serve Hot:

Serve the Whole Wheat Pasta with Chicken and Sun-Dried Tomatoes hot, savouring the rich flavours and textures.

Enjoy:

Enjoy a delightful and nutritious meal that brings together the goodness of whole wheat pasta, tender chicken, and vibrant Mediterranean ingredients.

Note: Feel free to customize the recipe by adding spinach or arugula for extra freshness or drizzling with a bit of extra olive oil before serving.

Nutrition Information (Per Serving):

• Calories: Approximately 400-450 calories

• Protein: 25g

• Carbohydrates: 45g

• Dietary Fiber: 8g

- Sugars: 4g
- Fat: 15g
- Saturated Fat: 4g
- Cholesterol: 60mg
- Sodium: 400mg

QUINOA AND CHICKPEA STUFFED BELL PEPPERS

Description: Experience a burst of flavours and textures with these Quinoa and chickpea-stuffed bell Peppers. This wholesome and protein-packed dish combines the nutty goodness of quinoa, chickpeas' heartiness, and bell peppers' vibrant colours. This vegetarian recipe is delicious and a feast for the eyes. Elevate your dinner table with these stuffed peppers, perfect for a nutritious and satisfying meal.

Ingredients:

For the Stuffed Bell Peppers:

• Four large bell peppers (any colour)

• 1 cup quinoa, cooked according to package instructions

• One can (15 oz) chickpeas, drained and rinsed

• 1 cup cherry tomatoes, diced

• 1/2 red onion, finely chopped

• Two cloves garlic, minced

• One teaspoon of ground cumin

• One teaspoon of smoked paprika

• Salt and black pepper to taste

• 1 cup shredded mozzarella or feta cheese (optional)

• Fresh parsley or cilantro for garnish

For the Sauce:

• One can (15 oz) tomato sauce

• One teaspoon dried oregano

• 1/2 teaspoon garlic powder

• Salt and black pepper to taste

Instructions:

Preheat Oven:

Preheat the oven to 375°F (190°C).

Prepare Bell Peppers:

Cut the tops off the bell peppers and remove the seeds and membranes. If needed, slice a small portion off the bottom to help them stand upright in the baking dish.

Prepare Quinoa and Chickpea Mixture:

Combine cooked quinoa, chickpeas, diced cherry tomatoes, chopped red onion, minced garlic, ground cumin, smoked paprika, salt, and black pepper in a large bowl. Mix well.

Stuff Bell Peppers:

Stuff each bell pepper with the quinoa and chickpea mixture. Press down gently to pack the filling.

Prepare Sauce:

Mix tomato sauce, dried oregano, garlic powder,

salt, and black pepper in a bowl. Pour the sauce over the stuffed peppers.

Bake:

Place the stuffed peppers in a baking dish. Cover with aluminium foil and bake in the preheated oven for 30-35 minutes or until the peppers are tender.

Optional Cheese Topping:

If using cheese, uncover the peppers, sprinkle shredded mozzarella or feta cheese on top, and bake for an additional 10 minutes or until the cheese is melted and bubbly.

Garnish and Serve:

Garnish the Quinoa and Chickpea Stuffed Bell Peppers with fresh parsley or cilantro. Serve hot.

Enjoy:

Enjoy a delightful and nutritious meal, savouring the combination of quinoa, chickpeas, and flavorful spices.

Note: Customize the recipe by adding your favourite vegetables or herbs to the quinoa and chickpea mixture for added freshness.

Nutrition Information (Per Serving):

• Calories: Approximately 300-350 calories

• Protein: 15g

• Carbohydrates: 50g

• Dietary Fiber: 8g

• Sugars: 8g

- Fat: 5g
- Saturated Fat: 2g
- Cholesterol: 10mg
- Sodium: 500mg

SUNFLOWER SEED AND BROCCOLI SALAD

Description: Indulge in the crisp and refreshing flavours of this Sunflower Seed and Broccoli Salad—a delightful combination of crunchy broccoli, sunflower seeds, and a zesty dressing. This vibrant salad is a feast for the senses and a nutritious addition to any meal. Whether served as a side dish or a light lunch, this recipe celebrates the simplicity of fresh ingredients while offering a burst of wholesome goodness.

Ingredients:

For the Salad:

- 4 cups broccoli florets, blanched

- 1/2 cup sunflower seeds, toasted

- 1/4 cup red onion, finely chopped

- 1/4 cup dried cranberries or raisins

- 1/4 cup feta cheese, crumbled (optional)

For the Dressing:

- 1/4 cup olive oil

- Two tablespoons of apple cider vinegar

- One tablespoon of honey or maple syrup

- One teaspoon of Dijon mustard

- Salt and black pepper to taste

Instructions:

Blanch Broccoli:

Bring a pot of water to a boil and blanch the broccoli florets for 1-2 minutes until they are bright green but still crisp. Immediately transfer them to a bowl of ice water to stop cooking. Drain and set aside.

Toast Sunflower Seeds:

Over medium heat, toast the sunflower seeds in a dry skillet until they become golden and fragrant. Be attentive to prevent burning. Set aside to cool.

Prepare Salad Base:

In a large salad bowl, combine the blanched broccoli, toasted sunflower seeds, finely chopped red onion, dried cranberries or raisins, and crumbled feta cheese if using.

Make the Dressing:

Whisk together olive oil, apple cider vinegar, honey or maple syrup, Dijon mustard, salt, and black pepper in a small bowl. Adjust the sweetness and acidity to your liking.

Toss and Coat:

Pour the dressing over the salad and toss gently to ensure all ingredients are coated evenly with the dressing.

Chill (Optional):

If time allows, let the salad chill in the refrigerator for 30 minutes to allow the flavours to meld.

Serve:

Serve the Sunflower Seed and Broccoli Salad as a refreshing or light lunch dish.

Enjoy:

Enjoy this delightful salad's crisp texture and vibrant flavours, embracing the wholesome combination of broccoli, sunflower seeds, and sweet-tangy dressing.

Note: Customize the salad by adding other ingredients such as cherry tomatoes, cucumber, or avocado for extra freshness.

Nutrition Information (Per Serving):

• Calories: Approximately 200-250 calories

• Protein: 5g

• Carbohydrates: 20g

• Dietary Fiber: 5g

• Sugars: 10g

• Fat: 15g

• Saturated Fat: 2g

• Cholesterol: 5mg

• Sodium: 150mg

PORK AND SWEET POTATO SKEWERS

Description: Savor the perfect balance of sweet and savoury with these Pork and Sweet Potato Skewers—a delicious combination of tender pork chunks and roasted sweet potato cubes threaded onto skewers. Infused with flavorful seasonings and grilled to perfection, this recipe is a delightful way to enjoy pork's succulence paired with sweet potatoes' natural sweetness. Elevate your grilling experience with these skewers that are easy to make and a crowd-pleaser.

Ingredients:

For the Skewers:

• 1.5 lbs pork loin or pork tenderloin, cut into cubes

• Two medium-sized sweet potatoes peeled and cut into cubes

• One red onion, cut into chunks

• Wooden or metal skewers, soaked if wooden

For the Marinade:

• 1/4 cup soy sauce

• Two tablespoons of olive oil

• Two tablespoons of honey or maple syrup

- Two cloves garlic, minced

- One teaspoon of smoked paprika

- One teaspoon of dried thyme

- Salt and black pepper to taste

Instructions:

Prepare Marinade:

Whisk together soy sauce, olive oil, honey or maple syrup, minced garlic, smoked paprika, dried thyme, salt, and black pepper in a bowl.

Marinate Pork:

Place the pork cubes in a resealable bag or shallow dish. Pour the marinade over the pork, ensuring each piece is coated. Marinate in the refrigerator for at least 30 minutes or a few hours for enhanced flavour.

Preheat Grill:

Preheat your grill to medium-high heat.

Prepare Sweet Potatoes:

Parboil the sweet potato cubes in boiling water for about 5 minutes or until slightly tender. Drain and let them cool slightly.

Assemble Skewers:

Thread marinated pork cubes, sweet potato cubes, and chunks of red onion onto the skewers, alternating for a colourful presentation.

Grill Skewers:

Place the assembled skewers on the preheated grill. Grill for 10-15 minutes, turning occasionally, until the pork is cooked through and the sweet potatoes are caramelized and tender.

Baste (Optional):

Optionally, baste the skewers with any remaining marinade during the grilling process for extra flavour.

Serve:

Once cooked, transfer the Pork and Sweet Potato Skewers to a serving platter.

Enjoy:

Enjoy the succulent pork, the sweetness of grilled sweet potatoes, and the savoury aroma of this delicious skewer recipe.

Note: Serve these skewers with a side of your favourite dipping sauce or a squeeze of fresh lemon for added brightness.

Nutrition Information (Per Serving):

• Calories: Approximately 300-350 calories

• Protein: 25g

• Carbohydrates: 20g

• Dietary Fiber: 3g

• Sugars: 8g

• Fat: 15g

• Saturated Fat: 4g

• Cholesterol: 70mg

• Sodium: 500mg

BROWN RICE AND BLACK BEAN BOWL

Description: Embrace a wholesome and nutritious meal with this Brown Rice and Black Bean Bowl—a flavorful combination of fibre-rich brown rice, protein-packed black beans, and vibrant vegetables. This easy-to-assemble bowl is delicious and versatile, allowing you to customize it with your favourite toppings and sauces. Enjoy a hearty and satisfying dish that brings together the goodness of whole grains, legumes, and fresh ingredients.

Ingredients:

For the Bowl:

• 2 cups cooked brown rice

• One can (15 oz) black beans, drained and rinsed

• 1 cup corn kernels (fresh, frozen, or canned)

• 1 cup cherry tomatoes, halved

• One avocado, sliced

• Fresh cilantro or parsley for garnish

• Lime wedges for serving

For the Dressing:

• Two tablespoons of olive oil

- One tablespoon of lime juice
- One teaspoon of ground cumin
- One teaspoon of chilli powder
- Salt and black pepper to taste

Instructions:

Prepare Brown Rice:

Cook brown rice according to package instructions. Fluff with a fork and set aside.

Make Dressing:

Whisk together olive oil, lime juice, ground cumin, chilli powder, salt, and black pepper in a small bowl to create the dressing.

Assemble the Bowl:

Layer cooked brown rice, black beans, corn kernels, cherry tomatoes, and avocado slices in serving bowls.

Drizzle with Dressing:

Drizzle the prepared dressing over the ingredients in the bowl.

Garnish:

Garnish the Brown Rice and Black Bean Bowl with fresh cilantro or parsley.

Serve with Lime Wedges:

Serve the bowls with lime wedges on the side for a burst of citrus flavour.

Customize (Optional):

Customize your bowl by adding ingredients like

diced red onion, bell peppers, or a dollop of Greek yoghurt.

Mix and Enjoy:

Toss the ingredients in the bowl gently to combine everything. Enjoy this wholesome and flavorful Brown Rice and Black Bean Bowl.

Note: Feel free to add your favourite hot sauce or salsa for an extra kick of flavour.

Nutrition Information (Per Serving):

• Calories: Approximately 400-450 calories

• Protein: 12g

• Carbohydrates: 60g

• Dietary Fiber: 12g

• Sugars: 4g

• Fat: 15g

• Saturated Fat: 2g

• Cholesterol: 0mg

• Sodium: 300mg

CAULIFLOWER AND WALNUT TACOS

Description: Experience a burst of flavours and textures with these Cauliflower and Walnut Tacos—a delicious and satisfying alternative to traditional meat-based tacos. Roasted cauliflower and toasted walnuts create a hearty and savoury filling, while a medley of fresh toppings adds a burst of freshness. Elevate your taco night with this plant-based recipe that's sure to become a new family favourite.

Ingredients:

For the Cauliflower and Walnut Filling:

• One medium cauliflower, cut into small florets

• 1 cup walnuts, finely chopped

• Two tablespoons of olive oil

• One teaspoon of ground cumin

• One teaspoon of smoked paprika

• 1/2 teaspoon chilli powder

• Salt and black pepper to taste

For the Tacos:

• Eight small corn or flour tortillas

• 1 cup shredded red cabbage

- One avocado, sliced
- Fresh cilantro, chopped
- Lime wedges for serving

For the Lime Crema:

- 1/2 cup Greek yoghurt or sour cream
- One tablespoon of lime juice
- One teaspoon lime zest
- Salt to taste

Instructions:

Preheat Oven:

Preheat the oven to 400°F (200°C).

Prepare Cauliflower and Walnut Filling:

In a large bowl, toss cauliflower florets and chopped walnuts with olive oil, ground cumin, smoked paprika, chilli powder, salt, and black pepper until well coated.

Roast:

Spread the cauliflower and walnut mixture on a baking sheet in a single layer. Roast in the oven for 20-25 minutes or until the cauliflower is golden and tender, stirring halfway through.

Prepare Lime Crema:

Whisk together Greek yoghurt or sour cream, lime juice, zest, and salt in a small bowl to create the lime crema. Adjust the seasoning to taste.

Warm Tortillas:

While the cauliflower and walnuts are roasting,

warm the tortillas in a dry skillet or in the oven according to package instructions.

Assemble Tacos:

Spoon the roasted cauliflower and walnut filling onto each tortilla. Top with shredded red cabbage, sliced avocado, and chopped cilantro.

Drizzle with Lime Crema:

Drizzle the tacos with the prepared lime crema.

Serve with Lime Wedges:

Serve the Cauliflower and Walnut Tacos with lime wedges on the side for an extra burst of citrus flavour.

Enjoy:

Enjoy these flavorful and satisfying plant-based tacos, embracing the goodness of roasted cauliflower and toasted walnuts.

Note: For extra flavour, customize your tacos with additional toppings such as salsa, diced tomatoes, or hot sauce.

Nutrition Information (Per Serving, 2 Tacos):

• Calories: Approximately 350-400 calories

• Protein: 10g

• Carbohydrates: 35g

• Dietary Fiber: 8g

• Sugars: 3g

• Fat: 20g

• Saturated Fat: 2g

- Cholesterol: 0mg
- Sodium: 300mg

CHAPTER SIX

Fatty Fish Recipes

Grilled Salmon with Lemon and Dill

Description: Indulge in a light and flavorful dish with this Grilled Salmon with Lemon and Dill—a simple yet elegant recipe that showcases the natural richness of salmon enhanced by the bright flavours of lemon and dill. The combination of grilling and zesty seasonings creates a perfect balance, making this salmon dish a delightful addition to your repertoire of healthy and delicious meals.

Ingredients:

For the Grilled Salmon:

• Four salmon fillets, skin-on

• Two tablespoons of olive oil

• Salt and black pepper to taste

• One lemon, sliced for garnish

• Fresh dill sprigs for garnish

For the Lemon-Dill Marinade:

• Juice of 1 lemon

• Zest of 1 lemon

• Two tablespoons fresh dill, chopped

• Two cloves garlic, minced

• One tablespoon of Dijon mustard

• Two tablespoons of olive oil

• Salt and black pepper to taste

Instructions:

Prepare Lemon-Dill Marinade:

Whisk together lemon juice, lemon zest, chopped fresh dill, minced garlic, Dijon mustard, olive oil, salt, and black pepper to create the marinade.

Marinate Salmon:

Place the salmon fillets in a shallow dish and pour the lemon-dill marinade over them. Ensure the fillets are well-coated. Allow them to marinate in the refrigerator for at least 30 minutes.

Preheat Grill:

Preheat your grill to medium-high heat.

Prepare Salmon for Grilling:

Remove the salmon fillets from the marinade and let any excess marinade drip off. Pat the fillets dry with a paper towel. Season both sides with salt and black pepper.

Grill Salmon:

Place the salmon fillets on the preheated grill, skin-side down. Grill for 4-5 minutes per side or until the salmon is cooked through and quickly flakes with a fork. The skin should be crispy.

Serve:

Transfer the grilled salmon to a serving platter. Garnish with lemon slices and fresh dill sprigs.

Enjoy:

Enjoy the Grilled Salmon with Lemon and Dill, savouring the perfectly grilled fish's delicate flavours and tender texture.

Note: Serve the grilled salmon alongside your favourite side dishes, such as quinoa, roasted vegetables, or a fresh green salad.

Nutrition Information (Per Serving):

• Calories: Approximately 300-350 calories

• Protein: 30g

• Carbohydrates: 2g

• Dietary Fiber: 0g

• Sugars: 0g

• Fat: 20g

• Saturated Fat: 3g

• Cholesterol: 80mg

• Sodium: 70mg

TUNA AND AVOCADO LETTUCE WRAPS

Description: Enjoy a light and refreshing meal with these Tuna and Avocado Lettuce Wraps—a healthy and flavorful option that combines the protein-rich goodness of tuna with the creamy texture of avocado. These wraps are delicious and low in carbohydrates, making them a perfect choice for a quick and satisfying lunch or dinner. Embrace the simplicity of fresh ingredients with this easy-to-make recipe.

Ingredients:

For the Tuna and Avocado Filling:

• Two cans (5 oz each) of tuna, drained

• One ripe avocado, diced

• 1/4 cup red onion, finely chopped

• 1/4 cup celery, finely chopped

• Two tablespoons fresh cilantro, chopped

• Two tablespoons mayonnaise

• One tablespoon of Dijon mustard

• Salt and black pepper to taste

- Juice of 1 lime

For the Lettuce Wraps:

- Large lettuce leaves (iceberg or butter lettuce work well)

Instructions:

Prepare Tuna and Avocado Filling:

Combine drained tuna, diced avocado, finely chopped red onion, celery, fresh cilantro, mayonnaise, Dijon mustard, salt, black pepper, and lime juice in a bowl. Mix gently until well combined.

Assemble Lettuce Wraps:

Spoon the tuna and avocado filling onto large lettuce leaves evenly.

Wrap and Serve:

Carefully fold the lettuce leaves around the filling to create wraps. Secure with toothpicks if needed.

Serve and Enjoy:

Arrange the Tuna and Avocado Lettuce Wraps on a platter and serve immediately. Enjoy the light and satisfying combination of tuna and creamy avocado.

Note: Customize the filling by adding ingredients like cherry tomatoes, cucumbers, or a dash of hot sauce for extra flavour.

Nutrition Information (Per Serving):

- Calories: Approximately 250-300 calories

- Protein: 20g

- Carbohydrates: 5g

- Dietary Fiber: 3g
- Sugars: 1g
- Fat: 18g
- Saturated Fat: 3g
- Cholesterol: 30mg
- Sodium: 400mg

MACKEREL AND QUINOA SALAD

Description: Indulge in a nutritious and flavorful Mackerel and Quinoa Salad—a delightful blend of protein-rich mackerel, wholesome quinoa, and an assortment of fresh vegetables. This salad is packed with omega-3 fatty acids and provides a satisfying and delicious combination of textures and flavours. Elevate your salad game with this easy-to-make recipe that's perfect for a light and wholesome meal.

Ingredients:

For the Salad:

- 1 cup cooked quinoa, cooled

- Two cans (about 7 oz each) of mackerel fillets, drained and flaked

- 1 cup cherry tomatoes, halved

- One cucumber, diced

- 1/4 cup red onion, finely chopped

- 1/4 cup Kalamata olives, sliced

- Two tablespoons fresh parsley, chopped

- Feta cheese crumbles for garnish (optional)

For the Lemon-Dill Vinaigrette:

- Three tablespoons olive oil
- Juice of 1 lemon
- One teaspoon of Dijon mustard
- One teaspoon of honey or maple syrup
- One teaspoon of fresh dill chopped
- Salt and black pepper to taste

Instructions:

Prepare Quinoa:

Cook quinoa according to package instructions. Once cooked, let it cool to room temperature.

Prepare Lemon-Dill Vinaigrette:

Whisk together olive oil, lemon juice, Dijon mustard, honey or maple syrup, fresh dill, salt, and black pepper in a small bowl to create the vinaigrette. Adjust the seasoning to taste.

Assemble Salad:

Combine cooled quinoa, flaked mackerel, cherry tomatoes, diced cucumber, finely chopped red onion, sliced Kalamata olives, and fresh parsley in a large salad bowl.

Drizzle with Vinaigrette:

Drizzle the lemon-dill vinaigrette over the salad ingredients. Toss gently to ensure an even coating.

Garnish with Feta (Optional):

Garnish the Mackerel and Quinoa Salad with feta cheese crumbles for an extra layer of flavour.

Serve and Enjoy:

Serve the salad immediately, enjoying the blend of textures and flavours from the mackerel, quinoa, and vibrant vegetables.

Note: Customize the salad by adding additional vegetables such as bell peppers, avocado, or arugula for extra freshness.

Nutrition Information (Per Serving):

• Calories: Approximately 350-400 calories

• Protein: 20g

• Carbohydrates: 25g

• Dietary Fiber: 4g

• Sugars: 3g

• Fat: 20g

• Saturated Fat: 3g

• Cholesterol: 40mg

• Sodium: 500mg

SMOKED SALMON AND CREAM CHEESE BAGEL

Description: Indulge in a classic and delicious breakfast or brunch with a Smoked Salmon and Cream Cheese Bagel—a timeless combination of flavours that showcases the rich taste of smoked salmon and the creamy texture of cream cheese. This easy-to-make recipe is a favourite for a reason, offering a perfect balance of savoury and tangy elements. Elevate your morning with this iconic dish that's both satisfying and luxurious.

Ingredients:

For the Bagel:

• One everything bagel, sliced and toasted

For the Toppings:

• 4 ounces smoked salmon

• Four tablespoons cream cheese (whipped or regular)

• Red onion, thinly sliced

• Capers drained

• Fresh dill for garnish

• Lemon wedges for serving

Instructions:

Toast the Bagel:

Slice the whole bagel and toast it until golden brown.

Spread Cream Cheese:

Spread a generous layer of cream cheese on each half of the toasted bagel.

Layer with Smoked Salmon:

Lay slices of smoked salmon evenly over the cream cheese on both halves of the bagel.

Add Toppings:

Top the smoked salmon with thinly sliced red onion and a sprinkle of capers.

Garnish with Fresh Dill:

Garnish the Smoked Salmon and Cream Cheese Bagel with fresh dill for a burst of herbaceous flavour.

Serve with Lemon Wedges:

Serve the bagel open-faced with lemon wedges on the side for a citrusy touch.

Enjoy:

Enjoy this classic Smoked Salmon and Cream Cheese Bagel for a luxurious and satisfying breakfast or brunch.

Note: Customize your bagel by adding additional toppings such as cucumber slices, arugula, or a sprinkle of black pepper for extra flavour.

Nutrition Information (Per Serving):

- Calories: Approximately 400-450 calories
- Protein: 20g
- Carbohydrates: 40g
- Dietary Fiber: 3g
- Sugars: 3g
- Fat: 20g
- Saturated Fat: 9g
- Cholesterol: 40mg
- Sodium: 800mg

CODFISH TACOS WITH MANGO SALSA

Description: Embark on a culinary journey with these Codfish Tacos with Mango Salsa—a delightful fusion of flaky codfish, vibrant mango salsa, and flavorful toppings encased in soft tortillas. This recipe combines the best fresh seafood and tropical fruits, creating a burst of colours and flavours perfect for a light and refreshing meal. Elevate your taco night with this easy-to-make and palate-pleasing dish.

Ingredients:

For the Codfish:

- 1 lb cod fillets

- Two tablespoons of olive oil

- One teaspoon of ground cumin

- One teaspoon of chilli powder

- 1/2 teaspoon garlic powder

- Salt and black pepper to taste

- Eight small flour or corn tortillas warmed

For the Mango Salsa:

- One ripe mango, diced
- 1/2 red onion, finely chopped
- One jalapeño, seeded and finely chopped
- 1/4 cup fresh cilantro, chopped
- Juice of 1 lime
- Salt to taste

For Toppings:

- Shredded cabbage or lettuce
- Avocado slices
- Greek yoghurt or sour cream
- Lime wedges for serving

Instructions:

Prepare Codfish:

Mix olive oil, ground cumin, chilli powder, garlic powder, salt, and black pepper in a bowl. Brush the cod fillets with the spice mixture, ensuring they are well coated.

Cook Codfish:

Heat a skillet over medium-high heat. Cook the cod fillets for 3-4 minutes per side or until they easily flake with a fork. Set aside.

Prepare Mango Salsa:

Combine diced mango, finely chopped red onion, jalapeño, cilantro, lime juice, and salt in a separate bowl. Mix well to create the mango salsa.

Assemble Tacos:

Flake the cooked cod into bite-sized pieces. Fill

each tortilla with flaked cod, shredded cabbage or lettuce, mango salsa, and avocado slices.

Add Toppings:

Drizzle with Greek yoghurt or sour cream, and add additional toppings like lime wedges if desired.

Serve and Enjoy:

Serve the Codfish Tacos with Mango Salsa immediately, savouring the combination of tender cod, sweet and spicy mango salsa, and fresh toppings.

Note: Customize the tacos with your favourite toppings, such as diced tomatoes, radishes, or a sprinkle of cotija cheese for added flavour.

Nutrition Information (Per Serving, 2 Tacos):

• Calories: Approximately 350-400 calories

• Protein: 20g

• Carbohydrates: 40g

• Dietary Fiber: 5g

• Sugars: 8g

• Fat: 15g

• Saturated Fat: 2g

• Cholesterol: 50mg

• Sodium: 500mg

TROUT AND ALMOND PILAF

Description: Elevate your dinner experience with this Trout and Almond Pilaf—a delectable dish combining flaky trout, aromatic pilaf, and crunchy almonds. This recipe boasts a harmonious blend of textures and flavours, creating a wholesome and satisfying meal. Delight in the simplicity of cooking trout over a bed of fragrant pilaf, complemented by the nutty goodness of almonds. Discover a new favourite for your repertoire of delicious and nutritious meals.

Ingredients:

For the Trout:

• Four trout fillets, skin-on

• Two tablespoons of olive oil

• Salt and black pepper to taste

• One lemon, sliced for garnish

• Fresh parsley for garnish

For the Almond Pilaf:

• 1 cup long-grain white rice

• 2 cups chicken or vegetable broth

• 1/4 cup sliced almonds, toasted

- 1/4 cup finely chopped onion
- Two cloves garlic, minced
- One tablespoon of olive oil
- One teaspoon of ground cumin
- 1/2 teaspoon ground coriander
- Salt and black pepper to taste

Instructions:

Prepare Almond Pilaf:

In a saucepan, heat one tablespoon of olive oil over medium heat. Add finely chopped onion and minced garlic, sautéing until softened.

Add Rice and Spices:

Stir in the rice and continue to cook for 2-3 minutes, allowing the rice to be toast toasted. Add ground cumin, ground coriander, salt, and black pepper. Mix well.

Pour Broth:

Pour in the chicken or vegetable broth and bring the mixture to a boil. Reduce the heat to low, cover the saucepan, and simmer for 15-18 minutes or until the rice is tender and the liquid is absorbed.

Toast Almonds:

While the pilaf is cooking, toast the sliced almonds in a dry skillet over medium heat until golden brown and fragrant. Set aside.

Prepare Trout:

Season the trout fillets with salt and black pepper. Heat 2 tablespoons of olive oil over medium-high heat in a separate skillet. Place the trout fillets skin-side down and cook for 3-4 minutes per side or until the skin is crispy and the flesh is flaky.

Assemble Dish:

Serve the trout fillets over a bed of almond pilaf. Garnish with toasted almonds, lemon slices, and fresh parsley.

Serve and Enjoy:

Enjoy the Trout and Almond Pilaf, savouring the combination of tender fish, flavorful pilaf, and crunchy almonds.

Note: Customize the pilaf by adding chopped dried apricots or raisins for a touch of sweetness.

Nutrition Information (Per Serving):

• Calories: Approximately 400-450 calories

• Protein: 25g

• Carbohydrates: 40g

• Dietary Fiber: 2g

• Sugars: 1g

• Fat: 18g

• Saturated Fat: 3g

• Cholesterol: 50mg

• Sodium: 500mg

HONEY GLAZED SALMON WITH SESAME SEEDS

Description: Treat your taste buds to a delightful culinary experience with this Honey Glazed Salmon with Sesame Seeds—a perfect balance of sweet and savoury flavours that complement the richness of salmon. The succulent salmon fillets are coated in a glossy honey glaze, creating a caramelized exterior while maintaining the tender flakiness inside. The addition of sesame seeds provides a nutty crunch, enhancing the overall texture. Enjoy this easy-to-make yet elegant dish for a delicious and wholesome meal.

Ingredients:

For the Honey Glaze:

• 1/4 cup honey

• Two tablespoons of soy sauce

• One tablespoon of Dijon mustard

• One tablespoon of rice vinegar

• Two cloves garlic, minced

• One teaspoon of sesame oil

- One teaspoon of grated ginger
- Sesame seeds for garnish

For the Salmon:

- Four salmon fillets, skin-on
- Salt and black pepper to taste
- Two tablespoons of olive oil

Instructions:

Preheat Oven:

Preheat your oven to 400°F (200°C).

Prepare Honey Glaze:

In a bowl, whisk together honey, soy sauce, Dijon mustard, rice vinegar, minced garlic, sesame oil, and grated ginger to create the honey glaze.

Season Salmon:

Pat the salmon fillets dry with a paper towel. Season both sides with salt and black pepper.

Sear Salmon:

In an oven-safe skillet, heat olive oil over medium-high heat. Sear the salmon fillets, skin-side down, for 2-3 minutes until the skin is crispy.

Glaze Salmon:

Brush the honey glaze over the salmon fillets, ensuring they are evenly coated.

Transfer to Oven:

Transfer the skillet to the preheated oven and bake for 8-10 minutes or until the salmon is cooked through and flakes quickly.

Broil for Caramelization (Optional):

If desired, broil the salmon for an additional 1-2 minutes to achieve a caramelized exterior.

Garnish with Sesame Seeds:

Sprinkle sesame seeds over the glazed salmon fillets for added crunch and flavour.

Serve:

Serve the Honey Glazed Salmon with Sesame Seeds on a platter, drizzling any remaining glaze over the top.

Enjoy:

Enjoy the sweet and savoury perfection of the honey-glazed salmon with sesame seeds.

Note: Serve the salmon over a bed of steamed rice or with your favourite roasted vegetables for a complete and satisfying meal.

Nutrition Information (Per Serving):

• Calories: Approximately 350-400 calories

• Protein: 25g

• Carbohydrates: 20g

• Dietary Fiber: 0g

• Sugars: 18g

• Fat: 20g

• Saturated Fat: 3g

• Cholesterol: 70mg

• Sodium: 400mg

SARDINE AND TOMATO BRUSCHETTA

Description: Elevate your appetizer game with this Sardine and Tomato Bruschetta—a flavorful twist on the classic Italian dish. The combination of savoury sardines, juicy tomatoes, and aromatic herbs creates a delightful topping that's rich in omega-3 fatty acids and bursts with Mediterranean flavours. Whether you're hosting a gathering or looking for a quick and tasty snack, this bruschetta is sure to impress with its vibrant taste and healthy ingredients.

Ingredients:

For the Sardine and Tomato Topping:

- One can (about 4 oz) sardines in olive oil, drained
- 1 cup cherry tomatoes, diced
- 1/4 cup red onion, finely chopped
- Two tablespoons fresh parsley, chopped
- One clove of garlic, minced
- Two tablespoons extra-virgin olive oil
- Juice of 1 lemon

• Salt and black pepper to taste

For the Bruschetta Base:

• Baguette or Italian bread, sliced

• Olive oil for brushing

• Garlic clove, peeled (for rubbing on the bread)

Instructions:

Prepare Sardine and Tomato Topping:

Combine drained sardines, diced cherry tomatoes, finely chopped red onion, fresh parsley, minced garlic, extra-virgin olive oil, and lemon juice in a bowl. Season with salt and black pepper. Mix gently to combine.

Slice and Toast the Bread:

Preheat your oven broiler. Slice the baguette or Italian bread into 1/2-inch thick slices. Place the slices on a baking sheet, brush with olive oil, and broil until golden brown.

Rub with Garlic:

While the bread is still warm, rub each slice with the peeled garlic clove. This imparts a subtle garlic flavour to the bread.

Top with Sardine Mixture:

Spoon the sardine and tomato mixture generously over each toasted bread slice.

Garnish:

Garnish the Sardine and Tomato Bruschetta with additional chopped parsley for freshness.

Serve:

Arrange the bruschetta on a serving platter and serve immediately.

Enjoy:

Enjoy this Sardine and Tomato Bruschetta as a delicious and nutritious appetizer or snack.

Note: Customize the bruschetta by adding a balsamic glaze drizzle or capers sprinkle for extra flavour.

Nutrition Information (Per Serving, 2 Bruschetta):

• Calories: Approximately 150-200 calories

• Protein: 8g

• Carbohydrates: 15g

• Dietary Fiber: 2g

• Sugars: 1g

• Fat: 8g

• Saturated Fat: 1g

• Cholesterol: 15mg

• Sodium: 200mg

CHAPTER SEVEN

Fortified Foods Recipes

Fortified whole-grain waffles with Berries

Description: Start your day with a nutritious and delicious twist by indulging in these Fortified Whole Grain Waffles with Berries. These waffles are made with wholesome whole grains and fortified with essential nutrients, creating a breakfast that's both satisfying and packed with goodness. Topped with a vibrant assortment of fresh berries, this breakfast dish is a delightful combination of flavours and textures that will fuel your morning with energy.

Ingredients:

For the Fortified Whole Grain Waffles:

• 1 cup whole wheat flour

• 1 cup all-purpose flour

• Two tablespoons ground flaxseed

• Two tablespoons chia seeds

• One tablespoon of baking powder

• 1/2 teaspoon salt

• Two tablespoons of honey or maple syrup

• Two large eggs

• 1 3/4 cups milk (dairy or plant-based)

• 1/4 cup melted coconut oil or unsalted butter

• One teaspoon of vanilla extract

For the Berry Topping:

• 1 cup strawberries, sliced

- 1/2 cup blueberries

- 1/2 cup raspberries

- Maple syrup for drizzling (optional)

Instructions:

Preheat Waffle Iron:

Preheat your waffle iron according to the manufacturer's instructions.

Prepare Waffle Batter:

Whisk together whole wheat flour, all-purpose flour, ground flaxseed, chia seeds, baking powder, and salt in a large bowl.

Mix Wet Ingredients:

Whisk together honey or maple syrup, eggs, milk, melted coconut oil or butter, and vanilla extract in another bowl.

Combine Wet and Dry Ingredients:

Pour the wet ingredients into the dry ingredients and stir until just combined. Do not overmix; some lumps are okay.

Cook Waffles:

Lightly grease the waffle iron with cooking spray. Ladle the batter onto the hot waffle iron and cook according to the manufacturer's instructions until golden brown and crisp.

Prepare Berry Topping:

While the waffles are cooking, wash and slice the strawberries and prepare the other berries.

Assemble and Serve:

Once the waffles are ready, place them on serving plates. Top with the fresh berry mixture and drizzle with maple syrup if desired.

Enjoy:

Enjoy these Fortified Whole Grain Waffles with Berries as a wholesome and satisfying breakfast that provides a nutritious start to your day.

Note: Customize your waffles with additional toppings such as Greek yoghurt, chopped nuts, or a sprinkle of cinnamon for extra flavour.

Nutrition Information (Per Serving, 2 Waffles):

• Calories: Approximately 350-400 calories

• Protein: 10g

• Carbohydrates: 50g

• Dietary Fiber: 7g

• Sugars: 10g

• Fat: 15g

• Saturated Fat: 10g

• Cholesterol: 80mg

• Sodium: 400mg

FORTIFIED ALMOND MILK SMOOTHIE

Description: Kickstart your day with a nutritious and refreshing Fortified Almond Milk Smoothie. This smoothie offers the creamy goodness of almond milk and is fortified with essential nutrients, making it a wholesome and satisfying beverage. Packed with a blend of fruits, vegetables, and protein, this smoothie provides a boost of energy to fuel your morning or serve as a delightful snack. Enjoy the delicious taste and nutritional benefits of every sip.

Ingredients:

• 1 cup fortified almond milk

• 1/2 frozen banana

• 1/2 cup frozen berries (such as blueberries, strawberries, or raspberries)

• 1/2 cup spinach leaves (fresh or frozen)

• 1/2 small avocado

• One tablespoon of chia seeds

• One scoop of protein powder (plant-based or whey, as per preference)

- One tablespoon of almond butter

- Ice cubes (optional)

Instructions:

Add Ingredients to Blender:

Place fortified almond milk, frozen banana, frozen berries, spinach, avocado, chia seeds, protein powder, and almond butter in a blender.

Blend Until Smooth:

Blend the ingredients on high speed until smooth and creamy. If the smoothie is too thick, you can add more almond milk or water to reach your desired consistency.

Adjust Sweetness (Optional):

Taste the smoothie and, if needed, add a natural sweetener such as honey or maple syrup to adjust the sweetness.

Add Ice Cubes (Optional):

If you prefer a colder and icier smoothie, add a handful of ice cubes and blend again until well incorporated.

Pour and Serve:

Pour the Fortified Almond Milk Smoothie into a glass and serve immediately.

Enjoy:

Savour the refreshing and nutritious goodness of this Fortified Almond Milk Smoothie as a nourishing start to your day or a revitalizing snack.

Note: Customize the smoothie by adding other ingredients, such as Greek yoghurt, a handful of kale, or a splash of vanilla extract for additional flavour.

Nutrition Information (Approximate):

• Calories: Approximately 300-350 calories

• Protein: 15g

• Carbohydrates: 25g

• Dietary Fiber: 8g

• Sugars: 10g

• Fat: 18g

• Saturated Fat: 2g

• Cholesterol: 20mg

• Sodium: 200mg

FORTIFIED CEREAL PARFAIT WITH YOGURT AND BERRIES

Description: Elevate your breakfast routine with a Fortified Cereal Parfait featuring creamy yoghurt, crunchy fortified cereal, and a vibrant mix of fresh berries. This parfait offers a delightful combination of textures and flavours and provides essential nutrients to kickstart your day. Whether enjoyed as a wholesome breakfast or a satisfying snack, this parfait is a delicious and nutritious way to fuel your body with the goodness it needs.

Ingredients:

• 1 cup fortified whole-grain cereal

• 1 cup Greek yoghurt (unsweetened or flavoured, as per preference)

• 1/2 cup mixed berries (strawberries, blueberries, raspberries)

• One tablespoon of honey or maple syrup (optional)

• One tablespoon chopped nuts (such as almonds or

walnuts)

- One tablespoon of ground flaxseed or chia seeds
- Fresh mint leaves for garnish (optional)

Instructions:

Prepare Ingredients:

Gather the fortified whole grain cereal, Greek yoghurt, mixed berries, honey or maple syrup (optional), chopped nuts, and ground flaxseed or chia seeds.

Layer the Parfait:

Start by layering a portion of the fortified whole grain cereal in a glass or bowl at the bottom.

Add Yogurt Layer:

Spoon a layer of Greek yoghurt over the cereal.

Add Berries:

Add a layer of mixed berries on top of the yoghurt.

Repeat Layers:

Repeat the layers until you reach the top of the glass or bowl, finishing with a sprinkle of fortified whole-grain cereal on the top.

Drizzle with Honey (Optional):

If desired, drizzle honey or maple syrup over the top for added sweetness.

Sprinkle Nuts and Seeds:

Sprinkle chopped nuts and ground flaxseed or chia seeds over the parfait for extra crunch and nutritional benefits.

Garnish (Optional):

Garnish with fresh mint leaves for a touch of freshness.

Serve:

Serve the Fortified Cereal Parfait immediately and enjoy the delicious layers of goodness.

Mix and Enjoy:

Before eating, mix the layers to combine the textures and flavours. Enjoy your nutritious and delightful parfait!

Note: Customize the parfait with your favourite fruits, granola, or additional toppings for variety.

Nutrition Information (Approximate):

• Calories: Approximately 300-350 calories

• Protein: 15g

• Carbohydrates: 40g

• Dietary Fiber: 8g

• Sugars: 15g

• Fat: 10g

• Saturated Fat: 2g

• Cholesterol: 10mg

• Sodium: 200mg

FORTIFIED ORANGE JUICE AND SPINACH SMOOTHIE

Description: Revitalize your morning with a nutrient-packed Fortified Orange Juice and Spinach Smoothie. This vibrant and refreshing smoothie combines the tangy sweetness of orange juice with the green goodness of spinach, creating a delightful beverage that's rich in vitamins and minerals. Fortified with additional nutrients, this smoothie is a delicious way to start your day on a healthy note. Enjoy the burst of flavours and the nourishing benefits of every sip.

Ingredients:

• 1 cup fortified orange juice (with added vitamin D and calcium)

• 1 cup fresh spinach leaves

• One frozen banana

• 1/2 cup Greek yoghurt (unsweetened or flavoured)

• One tablespoon of chia seeds

• One tablespoon of honey or maple syrup (optional)

• Ice cubes (optional)

Instructions:

Gather Ingredients:

Prepare the fortified orange juice, fresh spinach leaves, a frozen banana, Greek yoghurt, chia seeds, honey or maple syrup (optional), and ice cubes.

Add to Blender:

Combine the fortified orange juice, fresh spinach leaves, frozen banana, Greek yoghurt, and chia seeds in a blender.

Blend Until Smooth:

Blend the ingredients on high speed until the smoothie reaches a creamy and smooth consistency. If the smoothie is too thick, you can add more orange juice or water to achieve your desired thickness.

Taste and Sweeten (Optional):

Taste the smoothie and, if desired, add honey or maple syrup to sweeten it according to your preference.

Add Ice Cubes (Optional):

If you prefer a colder and icier smoothie, add a handful of ice cubes and blend again until well incorporated.

Pour and Serve:

Pour the Fortified Orange Juice and Spinach Smoothie into a glass.

Garnish (Optional):

Garnish with a slice of orange or a sprinkle of chia

seeds for an extra touch.

Enjoy:

Enjoy this nutritious and refreshing smoothie as a delightful way to boost your vitamin intake and start your day with a burst of energy.

Note: For added flavour and nutritional benefits, experiment with additional ingredients, such as a scoop of protein powder or a handful of berries.

Nutrition Information (Approximate):

• Calories: Approximately 250-300 calories

• Protein: 8g

• Carbohydrates: 50g

• Dietary Fiber: 8g

• Sugars: 30g

• Fat: 5g

• Saturated Fat: 1g

• Cholesterol: 5mg

• Sodium: 50mg

FORTIFIED TOFU SCRAMBLE

Description: Experience a delicious and nutrient-packed breakfast with this Fortified Tofu Scramble. Packed with plant-based protein and fortified with essential nutrients, this savoury tofu scramble is a flavorful and wholesome alternative to traditional scrambled eggs. The addition of colourful vegetables and a blend of seasonings creates a satisfying and nutritious meal that's perfect for starting your day on a healthful note.

Ingredients:

• 1 block firm tofu, pressed and crumbled

• One tablespoon of olive oil

• 1/2 onion, diced

• One bell pepper chopped (any colour)

• 1 cup cherry tomatoes, halved

• 2 cups fresh spinach

• Two cloves garlic, minced

• 1/2 teaspoon turmeric powder

• 1/2 teaspoon cumin powder

• 1/4 teaspoon smoked paprika

• Salt and black pepper to taste

• Two tablespoons nutritional yeast (fortified)

• Fresh herbs (such as parsley or chives) for garnish

• Avocado slices for serving (optional)

Instructions:

Press and Crumble Tofu:

Press the tofu to remove excess water, then crumble it into small pieces.

Sauté Vegetables:

In a large skillet, heat olive oil over medium heat. Add diced onion and bell pepper, sautéing until softened.

Add Tofu and Seasonings:

Add the crumbled tofu to the skillet. Sprinkle turmeric powder, cumin powder, smoked paprika, salt, and black pepper over the tofu. Mix well to distribute the seasonings evenly.

Cook Tofu Mixture:

Cook the tofu mixture for 5-7 minutes, stirring occasionally, until it begins to brown.

Add Vegetables and Garlic:

Add cherry tomatoes, fresh spinach, and minced garlic to the skillet. Cook for an additional 2-3 minutes, allowing the vegetables to soften and the spinach to wilt.

Incorporate Nutritional Yeast:

Stir in nutritional yeast, ensuring it coats the tofu and vegetables evenly. This adds a cheesy flavour and provides additional nutrients.

Adjust Seasonings:

Taste the tofu scramble and adjust the seasonings if needed. Add more salt, pepper, or nutritional yeast according to your preference.

Garnish and Serve:

Garnish the Fortified Tofu Scramble with fresh herbs (such as parsley or chives). Serve with optional avocado slices.

Enjoy:

Enjoy this Fortified Tofu Scramble on its own or as a filling for breakfast burritos or wraps.

Note: Customize the scramble by adding your favourite vegetables or a sprinkle of your preferred herbs and spices.

Nutrition Information (Approximate):

• Calories: Approximately 250-300 calories

• Protein: 20g

• Carbohydrates: 15g

• Dietary Fiber: 5g

• Sugars: 3g

• Fat: 15g

• Saturated Fat: 2g

• Cholesterol: 0mg

• Sodium: 300mg

FORTIFIED WHOLE WHEAT PANCAKES WITH MAPLE SYRUP

Description: Indulge in a delightful breakfast with Fortified Whole Wheat Pancakes, a wholesome twist on the classic morning treat. These pancakes are made with whole wheat flour for added fibre and are fortified with essential nutrients, making them a nutritious choice to kickstart your day. Drizzle with maple syrup for a touch of sweetness, and enjoy the perfect combination of fluffy texture and wholesome goodness.

Ingredients:

• 1 cup whole wheat flour

• One tablespoon of ground flaxseed

• One tablespoon of chia seeds

• One tablespoon of baking powder

• 1/4 teaspoon salt

• 1 cup fortified milk (dairy or plant-based)

• One large egg

- Two tablespoons melted coconut oil or unsalted butter
- One tablespoon of honey or maple syrup
- One teaspoon of vanilla extract
- Maple syrup for serving
- Fresh berries for garnish (optional)

Instructions:

Prepare Dry Ingredients:

Whisk together whole wheat flour, ground flaxseed, chia seeds, baking powder, and salt in a mixing bowl.

Mix Wet Ingredients:

Whisk together fortified milk, egg, melted coconut oil or butter, honey or maple syrup, and vanilla extract in a separate bowl.

Combine Wet and Dry Ingredients:

Pour the wet ingredients into the dry ingredients and stir until just combined. The batter may have lumps but avoid overmixing.

Preheat Griddle or Pan:

Preheat a griddle or non-stick pan over medium heat. Lightly grease with cooking spray or a small amount of oil.

Scoop and Cook Pancakes:

Scoop 1/4 cup portions of batter onto the griddle or pan to form pancakes. Cook until bubbles form on the surface, then flip and cook the other side until golden brown.

Repeat:

Repeat the process until all the batter is used, adjusting the heat if necessary.

Serve:

Stack the Fortified Whole Wheat Pancakes on a plate. Drizzle with maple syrup and garnish with fresh berries if desired.

Enjoy:

Enjoy these nutritious and delicious pancakes as a hearty breakfast or brunch option.

Note: Customize your pancakes by adding ingredients like blueberries, sliced bananas, or chopped nuts to the batter before cooking.

Nutrition Information (Approximate per serving):

• Calories: Approximately 200-250 calories

• Protein: 6g

• Carbohydrates: 30g

• Dietary Fiber: 4g

• Sugars: 8g

• Fat: 8g

• Saturated Fat: 5g

• Cholesterol: 40mg

• Sodium: 400mg

FORTIFIED BREAKFAST BURRITO WITH EGGS AND VEGETABLES

Description: Start your day with a satisfying and nutrient-packed Fortified Breakfast Burrito. Filled with fluffy scrambled eggs and a variety of colourful vegetables and fortified with essential nutrients, this burrito is a delicious and wholesome way to fuel your morning. Rolled up in a warm whole wheat tortilla, it's a convenient and portable breakfast that ensures you get a nourishing start to your day.

Ingredients:

• Four large eggs, beaten

• One tablespoon of olive oil

• 1/2 onion, diced

• One bell pepper (any colour), diced

• 1 cup cherry tomatoes, halved

- 1 cup spinach leaves, chopped

- 1/2 teaspoon cumin powder

- Salt and black pepper to taste

- Four whole wheat tortillas (large)

- 1 cup fortified black beans (canned or cooked)

- 1/2 cup shredded fortified cheese (cheddar or your choice)

- Avocado slices for topping (optional)

- Fresh cilantro for garnish (optional)

- Salsa or hot sauce for serving (optional)

Instructions:

Sauté Vegetables:

In a skillet, heat olive oil over medium heat. Add diced onion and bell pepper, sautéing until softened.

Add Eggs and Seasonings:

Pour beaten eggs into the skillet. Sprinkle cumin powder, salt, and black pepper over the eggs. Scramble the eggs until fully cooked.

Incorporate Vegetables:

Add cherry tomatoes and chopped spinach to the eggs. Cook for 2-3 minutes until the vegetables are heated and the spinach is wilted.

Warm Tortillas:

Warm the whole wheat tortillas in the skillet or microwave.

Assemble Burritos:

Lay out the tortillas and divide the fortified black beans evenly among them. Spoon the egg and vegetable mixture over the beans.

Add Cheese and Toppings:

Sprinkle shredded fortified cheese over the eggs. If desired, add avocado slices and fresh cilantro.

Roll Up Burritos:

Fold in the sides of each tortilla and then roll it up tightly to create a burrito.

Serve:

Place the Fortified Breakfast Burritos seam-side down on a plate. Cut them in half if desired.

Garnish and Enjoy:

Garnish with additional cilantro and serve with salsa or hot sauce on the side. Enjoy your nutrient-rich breakfast!

Note: Customize the burritos by adding ingredients such as diced avocado, Greek yoghurt, or your favourite hot sauce for extra flavour.

Nutrition Information (Approximate per burrito):

• Calories: Approximately 400-450 calories

• Protein: 20g

• Carbohydrates: 40g

• Dietary Fiber: 8g

• Sugars: 4g

• Fat: 20g

• Saturated Fat: 6g

- Cholesterol: 210mg
- Sodium: 600mg

FORTIFIED GRANOLA BARS WITH NUTS AND SEEDS

Description: Enjoy a nutritious and energy-boosting snack with these Fortified Granola Bars packed with various nuts and seeds. These bars provide a satisfying crunch and are fortified with essential nutrients, making them a wholesome choice for a quick pick-me-up. Whether you're on the go or need a healthy snack, these homemade granola bars are a delicious way to fuel your body with the goodness of nuts, seeds, and fortifying ingredients.

Ingredients:

- 2 cups old-fashioned rolled oats

- 1 cup mixed nuts (almonds, walnuts, pecans), chopped

- 1/2 cup mixed seeds (sunflower seeds, pumpkin seeds, flaxseeds)

- 1/2 cup dried fruits (cranberries, raisins, apricots), chopped

- 1/2 cup honey or maple syrup

- 1/4 cup coconut oil
- 1/4 cup almond butter or peanut butter
- One teaspoon of vanilla extract
- 1/2 teaspoon cinnamon
- 1/4 teaspoon salt
- 1/2 cup fortified protein powder
- 1/4 cup dark chocolate chips (optional for drizzling)

Instructions:

Preheat Oven:

Preheat your oven to 350°F (175°C). Line a baking pan with parchment paper, leaving some overhang for easy removal.

Mix Dry Ingredients:

Combine rolled oats, chopped nuts, mixed seeds, and dried fruits in a large bowl. Mix well to distribute evenly.

Prepare Wet Ingredients:

Combine honey or maple syrup, coconut oil, almond butter or peanut butter, vanilla extract, cinnamon, and salt in a small saucepan over low heat. Stir until the mixture is well combined and smooth.

Combine Wet and Dry Ingredients:

Pour the wet ingredients over the dry ingredients. Mix thoroughly to ensure all the dry ingredients are coated with the wet mixture.

Add Protein Powder:

Fold in the fortified protein powder, ensuring it is evenly distributed throughout the mixture.

Press into Pan:

Transfer the mixture to the prepared baking pan. Press it down firmly and evenly to create a compact layer.

Bake:

Bake in the preheated oven for 20-25 minutes or until the edges are golden brown.

Cool and Cut:

Allow the granola bars to cool completely in the pan. Once cooled, lift the parchment paper to remove the slab and cut it into bars of your desired size.

Optional Chocolate Drizzle:

Melt dark chocolate chips and drizzle over the top of the bars for a decadent touch.

Store:

Store the Fortified Granola Bars in an airtight container at room temperature for up to a week, or refrigerate for a longer shelf life.

Note: Customize the granola bars by adding other ingredients such as shredded coconut, chia seeds, or dried berries for extra flavour and texture.

Nutrition Information (Approximate, per bar):

• Calories: Approximately 200-250 calories

• Protein: 8g

• Carbohydrates: 20g

- Dietary Fiber: 4g
- Sugars: 8g
- Fat: 12g
- Saturated Fat: 3g
- Cholesterol: 0mg
- Sodium: 50mg

CHAPTER EIGHT

Vitamin D Sources Recipes

Sun-Dried Tomato and Basil Omelette

Description: Elevate your breakfast with the delightful flavors of this Sun-Dried Tomato and Basil Omelette. Packed with the richness of sun-dried tomatoes and the freshness of basil, this omelette is a delicious and savoury way to start your day. Fortified with essential nutrients, it offers a wholesome and flavorful breakfast that's quick to prepare and guaranteed to satisfy your taste buds.

Ingredients:

• Three large eggs

• One tablespoon of olive oil

• Two tablespoons sun-dried tomatoes, chopped

• Two tablespoons fresh basil, thinly sliced

• 1/4 cup feta cheese, crumbled

• Salt and black pepper to taste

• 1/2 teaspoon dried oregano (optional)

• 1/4 cup fortified milk (dairy or plant-based)

• Cooking spray or additional olive oil for greasing

Instructions:

Whisk Eggs:

In a bowl, whisk the eggs until well combined. Add fortified milk, salt, and black pepper. Whisk again until the mixture is smooth.

Prep Ingredients:

Chop the sun-dried tomatoes, slice the fresh basil, and crumble the feta cheese.

Heat Olive Oil:

Heat olive oil in a non-stick skillet over medium heat.

Sauté Sun-Dried Tomatoes:

Add the chopped sun-dried tomatoes to the skillet and sauté for 1-2 minutes until they start to release their flavour.

Pour in Egg Mixture:

Pour the whisked egg mixture over the sautéed sun-dried tomatoes. Swirl the pan to ensure an even distribution.

Add Basil and Feta:

Sprinkle fresh basil and crumbled feta cheese over one-half of the omelette.

Fold and Cook:

Once the edges of the omelette begin to set, use a spatula to gently fold it in half, covering the basil and feta.

Cook Until Set:

Cook for an additional 1-2 minutes until the omelette is fully set but still moist.

Season and Garnish:

Season the omelette with dried oregano if desired. Garnish with additional fresh basil.

Serve:

Slide the Sun-Dried Tomato and Basil Omelette onto a plate and serve immediately.

Enjoy:

Enjoy this flavorful and fortified omelette as a satisfying breakfast or brunch option.

Note: Customize the omelette by adding other ingredients like sautéed mushrooms, spinach, or diced bell peppers for extra variety.

Nutrition Information (Approximate):

• Calories: Approximately 300-350 calories

• Protein: 20g

• Carbohydrates: 5g

• Dietary Fiber: 1g

• Sugars: 2g

• Fat: 24g

• Saturated Fat: 8g

• Cholesterol: 490mg

• Sodium: 400mg

GRILLED PORTOBELLO MUSHROOMS WITH EGG

Description: Indulge in a savoury and satisfying breakfast with this Grilled Portobello Mushrooms with Egg dish. Fortify your morning with the rich, umami flavour of grilled portobello mushrooms combined with a perfectly cooked egg. This hearty and nutritious dish provides a unique twist to your breakfast routine and offers a substantial dose of essential nutrients to kickstart your day.

Ingredients:

• Two large portobello mushrooms, stems removed

• Two eggs

• Two tablespoons of olive oil

• Two cloves garlic, minced

• One teaspoon of fresh thyme leaves

• Salt and black pepper to taste

• Fresh parsley for garnish (optional)

• Grated Parmesan cheese for topping (optional)

Instructions:

Prepare Portobello Mushrooms:

Clean the portobello mushrooms with a damp cloth. Remove the stems and gently scrape out the gills using a spoon.

Marinate Mushrooms:

Mix olive oil, minced garlic, fresh thyme leaves, salt, and black pepper in a small bowl. Brush this marinade over both sides of the portobello mushrooms.

Preheat Grill or Grill Pan:

Preheat a grill or grill pan over medium heat.

Grill Mushrooms:

Place the marinated portobello mushrooms on the preheated grill. Grill each side for 4-5 minutes or until tender.

Create Egg Pockets:

Once the mushrooms are grilled, crack an egg into the centre of each mushroom, making a pocket for the egg.

Grill Eggs:

Close the grill lid or cover the mushrooms with a lid or foil. Grill for an additional 5-7 minutes or until the eggs are cooked to your liking.

Season and Garnish:

Season the eggs with additional salt and black pepper if needed. Garnish with fresh parsley and grated Parmesan cheese if desired.

Serve:

Carefully transfer the Grilled Portobello Mushrooms with Egg to serving plates.

Enjoy:

Enjoy this flavorful and protein-packed breakfast with the delicious combination of grilled portobello mushrooms and a perfectly grilled egg.

Note: Customize the dish by adding your favourite herbs, spices, or toppings, such as diced tomatoes or avocado.

Nutrition Information (Approximate):

• Calories: Approximately 250-300 calories

• Protein: 15g

• Carbohydrates: 5g

• Dietary Fiber: 2g

• Sugars: 1g

• Fat: 20g

• Saturated Fat: 4g

• Cholesterol: 370mg

• Sodium: 150mg

SMOKED HERRING SALAD WITH AVOCADO

Description: Elevate your lunch with the rich flavours of this Smoked Herring Salad featuring creamy avocado. Packed with omega-3 fatty acids and vibrant ingredients, this salad offers a delightful combination of textures and tastes and provides a nutritious and satisfying meal. Enjoy the unique smokiness of herring paired with the buttery goodness of avocado in this delicious and fortifying salad.

Ingredients:

• 1 cup smoked herring fillets, flaked

• One ripe avocado, diced

• 1 cup cherry tomatoes, halved

• 1/4 red onion, thinly sliced

• Two tablespoons fresh cilantro, chopped

• One tablespoon extra-virgin olive oil

• One tablespoon of red wine vinegar

• One teaspoon of Dijon mustard

• Salt and black pepper to taste

- Mixed salad greens for serving (optional)

Instructions:

Prepare Herring and Vegetables:

Flake the smoked herring fillets into bite-sized pieces. Dice the ripe avocado, halve the cherry tomatoes, thinly slice the red onion, and chop the fresh cilantro.

Assemble Salad:

Combine the flaked smoked herring, diced avocado, halved cherry tomatoes, sliced red onion, and chopped cilantro in a large bowl.

Prepare Dressing:

Whisk together extra-virgin olive oil, red wine vinegar, Dijon mustard, salt, and black pepper in a small bowl to create the dressing.

Dress the Salad:

Pour the dressing over the salad ingredients. Gently toss the salad until everything is well-coated.

Serve on Greens (Optional):

For an extra boost of greens, serve the Smoked Herring Salad on a bed of mixed salad greens.

Adjust Seasonings:

Taste the salad and adjust the seasonings if needed, adding more salt, pepper, or a drizzle of olive oil according to your preference.

Serve Immediately:

Serve the Smoked Herring Salad with Avocado

immediately, enjoying the contrast of smoky herring, creamy avocado, and the freshness of other ingredients.

Enjoy:

Enjoy this flavorful and nutrient-rich salad as a light, satisfying lunch or dinner option.

Note: Customize the salad by adding ingredients like cucumber, radishes, or a squeeze of lemon juice for extra freshness.

Nutrition Information (Approximate):

• Calories: Approximately 300-350 calories

• Protein: 20g

• Carbohydrates: 15g

• Dietary Fiber: 7g

• Sugars: 3g

• Fat: 20g

• Saturated Fat: 3g

• Cholesterol: 35mg

• Sodium: 600mg

BAKED COD WITH LEMON AND HERBS

Description: Savor the delicate flavours of the sea with this light and refreshing Baked Cod with Lemon and Herbs. This dish highlights the natural taste of cod enhanced with zesty lemon and aromatic herbs. Quick to prepare and baked to perfection, this recipe offers a healthy and flavorful option for a delightful seafood dinner. Immerse yourself in the simplicity of fresh ingredients and the goodness of baked cod.

Ingredients:

• Four cod fillets (about 6 ounces each)

• Two tablespoons of olive oil

• Two tablespoons of fresh lemon juice

• Two cloves garlic, minced

• One teaspoon of fresh thyme leaves

• One teaspoon of fresh parsley chopped

• 1/2 teaspoon dried oregano

• Salt and black pepper to taste

• Lemon slices for garnish (optional)

• Fresh parsley for garnish (optional)

Instructions:

Preheat Oven:

Preheat your oven to 400°F (200°C).

Prepare Cod Fillets:

Pat the cod fillets dry with paper towels and place them in a baking dish.

Prepare Herb Mixture:

In a small bowl, combine olive oil, fresh lemon juice, minced garlic, fresh thyme leaves, chopped parsley, dried oregano, salt, and black pepper. Mix well to create the herb mixture.

Coat Cod Fillets:

Pour the herb mixture over the cod fillets, ensuring they are evenly coated on both sides.

Marinate (Optional):

Allow the cod to marinate for 15-20 minutes to let the flavours infuse.

Bake Cod:

Bake the cod fillets in the preheated oven for 12-15 minutes or until the fish flakes easily with a fork.

Broil (Optional):

If desired, broil the cod for an additional 2-3 minutes to achieve a golden brown colour on top.

Garnish and Serve:

Garnish the Baked Cod with Lemon and Herbs with lemon slices and fresh parsley.

Serve Immediately:

Serve the baked cod immediately, allowing the

vibrant flavours to shine.

Enjoy:

Enjoy this light and flavorful Baked Cod with Lemon and Herbs as a nutritious and satisfying main dish.

Note: Customize the dish by adding a sprinkle of red pepper flakes for a hint of heat or serving it with a side of roasted vegetables.

Nutrition Information (Approximate per serving):

• Calories: Approximately 200-250 calories

• Protein: 25g

• Carbohydrates: 2g

• Dietary Fiber: 1g

• Sugars: 0g

• Fat: 12g

• Saturated Fat: 2g

• Cholesterol: 60mg

• Sodium: 300mg

SAUTÉED SWISS CHARD WITH GARLIC AND SUNFLOWER SEEDS

Description: Elevate your greens with this vibrant and flavorful dish of Sautéed Swiss Chard with Garlic and Sunflower Seeds. Packed with nutrients and bursting with colour, this recipe transforms Swiss chard into a delightful side dish or a nutritious addition to your meal. The combination of garlic and sunflower seeds adds a savoury and crunchy element, making it a perfect complement to any main course.

Ingredients:

- One bunch of Swiss chard, washed and chopped
- Two tablespoons of olive oil
- Three cloves garlic, minced
- Two tablespoons sunflower seeds
- Salt and black pepper to taste
- Crushed red pepper flakes (optional, for a hint of spice)
- Lemon wedges for serving (optional)

Instructions:

Prepare Swiss Chard:

Wash the Swiss chard thoroughly, remove the stems, and chop the leaves into bite-sized pieces.

Sauté Garlic:

In a large skillet, heat olive oil over medium heat. Add minced garlic and sauté for about 1 minute until fragrant.

Add Swiss Chard:

Add the chopped Swiss chard to the skillet. Stir to coat the leaves with the garlic-infused oil.

Sauté Until Wilted:

Sauté the Swiss chard for 3-5 minutes or until the leaves are wilted and tender. Stir occasionally to ensure even cooking.

Add Sunflower Seeds:

Sprinkle sunflower seeds over the sautéed Swiss chard. Continue to cook for an additional 1-2 minutes, allowing the sunflower seeds to toast slightly.

Season:

Season the dish with salt, black pepper, and optional crushed red pepper flakes for a touch of heat. Adjust the seasoning to taste.

Serve:

Transfer the Sautéed Swiss Chard with Garlic and Sunflower Seeds to a serving dish.

Garnish and Serve:

Garnish with additional sunflower seeds and serve with lemon wedges on the side for a citrusy touch if desired.

Enjoy:

Enjoy this nutritious and flavorful side dish as a perfect accompaniment to your favourite protein or as a standalone dish.

Note: Experiment with different seeds or nuts for added texture and flavour, and consider finishing with a squeeze of fresh lemon juice for brightness.

Nutrition Information (Approximate per serving):

• Calories: Approximately 150-200 calories

• Protein: 5g

• Carbohydrates: 8g

• Dietary Fiber: 3g

• Sugars: 2g

• Fat: 12g

• Saturated Fat: 2g

• Cholesterol: 0mg

• Sodium: 300mg

SHIITAKE MUSHROOM AND TOFU STIR-FRY

Description: Experience a symphony of flavours and textures with this Shiitake Mushroom and Tofu Stir-Fry. Packed with umami from shiitake mushrooms and the protein goodness of tofu, this dish is a delightful and nutritious option for a quick and satisfying meal. The vibrant vegetables, savoury sauce, and tender tofu create a well-balanced stir-fry that will tantalize your taste buds.

Ingredients:

For the Stir-Fry:

• One block of firm tofu pressed and cubed

• 2 cups shiitake mushrooms, sliced

• One bell pepper, thinly sliced (any colour)

• One carrot, julienned

• 1 cup snow peas, ends trimmed

• Three green onions, sliced

• Two tablespoons of vegetable oil

For the Sauce:

- Three tablespoons soy sauce
- One tablespoon of hoisin sauce
- One tablespoon of rice vinegar
- One tablespoon of maple syrup or honey
- Two teaspoons of sesame oil
- Two cloves garlic, minced
- One teaspoon of fresh ginger, grated
- One teaspoon of cornstarch (optional for thickening)

For Garnish:

- Sesame seeds
- Chopped cilantro or parsley

Instructions:

Prepare Tofu:

Press the tofu to remove excess water, then cube it into bite-sized pieces.

Make Sauce:

Whisk together soy sauce, hoisin sauce, rice vinegar, maple syrup or honey, sesame oil, minced garlic, and grated ginger in a small bowl. If you prefer a thicker sauce, add cornstarch and mix well.

Stir-Fry Tofu:

Heat one tablespoon of vegetable oil in a wok or large skillet over medium-high heat. Add the cubed tofu and cook until all sides are golden brown. Remove tofu from the pan and set aside.

Sauté Vegetables:

In the same pan, add another tablespoon of vegetable oil. Add shiitake mushrooms, bell pepper, julienned carrot, and snow peas. Stir-fry for 3-4 minutes until the vegetables are crisp-tender.

Combine Tofu and Sauce:

Return the cooked tofu to the pan with the vegetables. Pour the sauce over the tofu and vegetables. Stir to coat everything evenly.

Finish Cooking:

Cook for an additional 2-3 minutes until the sauce thickens slightly and the tofu and vegetables are well-coated.

Add Green Onions:

Stir in sliced green onions during the last minute of cooking.

Garnish and Serve:

Garnish the Shiitake Mushroom and Tofu. Stir-fry with sesame seeds and chopped cilantro or parsley.

Serve Over Rice or Noodles:

Serve the stir-fry over cooked rice or noodles.

Enjoy:

Enjoy this flavorful and nutrient-packed Shiitake Mushroom and Tofu Stir-Fry as a delicious and wholesome meal.

Note: Customize the stir-fry by adding your favourite vegetables or adjusting the sauce ingredients to suit your taste.

Nutrition Information (Approximate per serving):

• Calories: Approximately 300-350 calories

• Protein: 15g

• Carbohydrates: 20g

• Dietary Fiber: 5g

• Sugars: 8g

• Fat: 20g

• Saturated Fat: 3g

• Cholesterol: 0mg

• Sodium: 700mg

VITAMIN D-ENRICHED MUSHROOM SOUP

Description: Warm up with a comforting bowl of Vitamin D-enriched Mushroom Soup, a delightful blend of earthy mushrooms and nourishing ingredients. This soup offers the rich flavours of mushrooms and provides an extra boost of vitamin D for your well-being. Enjoy the wholesome goodness of this soup as a hearty appetizer or a light meal, perfect for any season.

Ingredients:

• 1 pound (450g) mixed mushrooms (such as cremini, shiitake, and button mushrooms), sliced

• One onion, finely chopped

• 2 cloves garlic, minced

• Two tablespoons of olive oil

• 4 cups vegetable or chicken broth (low-sodium)

• One medium potato, peeled and diced

• One carrot, peeled and diced

• One celery stalk, diced

• One teaspoon of dried thyme

- One teaspoon of dried rosemary

- One bay leaf

- Salt and black pepper to taste

- 1 cup Vitamin D-enriched milk (dairy or plant-based)

- Two tablespoons flour (all-purpose or gluten-free for thickening)

- Fresh parsley for garnish (optional)

Instructions:

Sauté Mushrooms:

In a large pot, heat olive oil over medium heat. Add chopped onions and minced garlic. Sauté until onions are translucent.

Add Mushrooms:

Add sliced mushrooms to the pot. Cook for 5-7 minutes until the mushrooms release their moisture and start to brown.

Prepare Vegetables:

Add diced potato, carrot, and celery to the pot. Stir well to combine.

Season:

Season the vegetables and mushrooms with dried thyme, dried rosemary, bay leaf, salt, and black pepper.

Add Broth:

Pour in the vegetable or chicken broth. Bring the mixture to a simmer and let it cook for 15-20 minutes until the vegetables are tender.

Thicken Soup:

Whisk together Vitamin D-enriched milk and flour in a separate bowl until smooth. Slowly pour this mixture into the soup, stirring constantly to prevent lumps. Simmer for an additional 5-7 minutes until the soup thickens.

Adjust Seasoning:

Taste the soup and adjust the seasoning if needed. Remove the bay leaf.

Serve:

Ladle the Vitamin D-enriched Mushroom Soup into bowls. Garnish with fresh parsley if desired.

Enjoy:

Enjoy this comforting and nutrient-rich soup as a wholesome appetizer or a light meal.

Note: Customize the soup by adding a dash of nutmeg or a squeeze of lemon juice for additional flavour.

Nutrition Information (Approximate per serving):

• Calories: Approximately 150-200 calories

• Protein: 5g

• Carbohydrates: 20g

• Dietary Fiber: 4g

• Sugars: 5g

• Fat: 7g

• Saturated Fat: 1g

• Cholesterol: 0mg

• Sodium: 600mg

BAKED EGGPLANT WITH TOMATO AND PARMESAN

Description: Indulge in the savoury goodness of this Baked Eggplant with Tomato and Parmesan, a delightful dish that brings together the robust flavours of ripe tomatoes, tender eggplant, and the richness of Parmesan cheese. This simple yet elegant recipe offers a satisfying combination of textures and tastes, making it a perfect side dish or a light vegetarian meal. Enjoy the wholesome goodness of baked eggplant infused with Mediterranean flavours.

Ingredients:

• Two medium-sized eggplants, sliced into rounds

• Two large tomatoes, thinly sliced

• 1 cup grated Parmesan cheese

• 1/4 cup fresh basil leaves, chopped

• Two cloves garlic, minced

• 1/4 cup olive oil

• Salt and black pepper to taste

• Balsamic glaze for drizzling (optional)

Instructions:

1. Preheat Oven:

• Preheat your oven to 400°F (200°C).

1. Prepare Eggplant:

• Slice the eggplants into rounds approximately 1/2-inch thick. Place the slices on a paper towel and sprinkle them with salt. Allow them to sit for 15-20 minutes to draw out excess moisture.

1. Pat Dry Eggplant:

• Pat the eggplant slices dry with a paper towel to remove the released moisture.

1. Arrange Eggplant in Baking Dish:

• In a baking dish, arrange the eggplant slices in a single layer.

1. Layer with Tomatoes:

• Place thinly sliced tomatoes over the eggplant rounds.

1. Combine Garlic, Basil, and Olive Oil:

• Mix minced garlic, chopped fresh basil, and olive oil in a small bowl.

1. Drizzle Olive Oil Mixture:

• Drizzle the olive oil mixture over the eggplant and tomatoes, ensuring they are well-coated.

1. Season and Add Parmesan:

• Season with salt and black pepper. Sprinkle-grated Parmesan cheese generously over the top.

1. Bake:

• Bake in the preheated oven for 20-25 minutes or until

the eggplant is tender and the Parmesan is golden and bubbly.

1. Broil (Optional):

• If desired, broil for an additional 2-3 minutes to achieve a golden brown crust on top.

1. Drizzle with Balsamic Glaze:

• Optionally, drizzle balsamic glaze over the baked eggplant for added flavour.

1. Serve:

• Serve the Baked Eggplant with Tomato and Parmesan as a delicious side dish or a light vegetarian main course.

1. Enjoy:

• Enjoy the rich and savoury flavours of this Mediterranean-inspired baked eggplant dish.

Note: Customize the recipe by adding a sprinkle of dried oregano or red pepper flakes for additional flavour.

Nutrition Information (Approximate per serving):

• Calories: Approximately 200-250 calories

• Protein: 10g

• Carbohydrates: 15g

• Dietary Fiber: 8g

• Sugars: 7g

• Fat: 15g

• Saturated Fat: 5g

• Cholesterol: 20mg

• Sodium: 400mg

CONCLUSION

In conclusion, the intricate interplay between osteoporosis and diet underscores the profound impact of nutritional choices on bone health. Osteoporosis, characterized by compromised bone density and increased vulnerability to fractures, demands a multifaceted approach to prevention and management. As we have explored, a well-balanced and nutrient-rich diet emerges as a cornerstone in this strategy, providing the essential building blocks for bone formation, maintenance, and resilience.

The significance of calcium, vitamin D, protein, phosphorus, magnesium, and vitamin K in maintaining optimal bone health cannot be overstated. These nutrients, derived from diverse foods, contribute synergistically to the intricate web of bone metabolism. While calcium forms the structural foundation of bones, vitamin D facilitates its absorption, and protein, phosphorus, magnesium, and vitamin K play complementary roles in bone density and strength.

Moreover, the broader lifestyle choices, such as limiting caffeine and alcohol intake, maintaining a low-sodium diet, and engaging in weight-bearing exercises, serve to reinforce the positive impact of a bone-healthy diet. As we navigate the complexities of osteoporosis, it is evident that a holistic approach encompassing dietary modifications, regular exercise, and lifestyle adjustments can significantly enhance bone integrity and reduce the risk of fractures.

As we strive for a comprehensive understanding of osteoporosis and its relationship with diet, it is essential to acknowledge the importance of individualized care. Recognizing that dietary needs may vary based on age, gender, genetics, and overall health status, consultation with healthcare professionals, notably registered dietitians, is paramount. Tailoring dietary recommendations to meet individual requirements ensures an approach that is both effective and sustainable.

In essence, the role of diet in osteoporosis extends beyond a mere dietary regimen; it embodies a proactive and empowering approach to skeletal health. By embracing a nutrient-dense diet, individuals can fortify their bones, enhancing their quality of life and mitigating the impact of osteoporosis. Through ongoing research, education, and personalized healthcare, we pave the way toward a future where the intersection of diet and bone health becomes a cornerstone in the prevention and management of osteoporosis.

www.ingramcontent.com/pod-product-compliance
Lightning Source LLC
Chambersburg PA
CBHW050726260726
48661CB00001B/79